DIETS STILL DON'T WORK!

How To Lose Weight Step-By-Step Even After You've Failed At Dieting

by Bob Schwartz
Author of the New York Times Best Seller,
DIETS DON'T WORK!,
and THE ONE HOUR ORGASM

DIETS STILL DON'T WORK!

First Printing   April 1990

Copyright© 1990 by Robert M. Schwartz

ISBN 0-942540-04-2
1 2 3 4 5 6 7 8 9 10/99 98 97 96 95 94 93 92 91 90

Published by
BREAKTHRU PUBLISHING
P.O. BOX 2866
Houston, Texas 77252–2866
(713) 522–7660

Printed in the United States of America

ACKNOWLEDGMENTS

I wish to thank the half million people who read my first book, *DIETS DON'T WORK*, and courageously used it to change their lives. Also to the thousands who participated in my Weekend Breakthru Workshops for Overeating and Weight Disorders, plus those who worked with me individually.

To Leah, my wife and love of my life, who lost 40 pounds from reading the manuscript of *DIETS DON'T WORK* and who has kept her weight off without dieting for 11 years.

Editor: Dr. Frank Reuter, Ph. D.
Typesetting: J. Jones of Word Merchant

PREFACE

DIETS STILL DON'T WORK is about many of
the new discoveries and breakthroughs gathered
over the last 8 years from many of the half
million readers of the New York Times Best
Seller *DIETS DON'T WORK*. *DIETS STILL DON'T
WORK* contains new information which will be
valuable to those who have already read Bob
Schwartz's first book, *DIETS DON'T WORK*, as
well as those who have not. Some of the logic
may be familiar to the reader of *DIETS DON'T
WORK*, but repetition is a valuable teacher. Much
of the information has also been updated to
clarify some fine points and to produce results
faster for readers.

Many questions which were often asked after
the reading of *DIETS DON'T WORK* have been
answered and clarified such as:

1. What to do when you <u>already</u> know what
to do, but aren't doing it.

2. How to beat the "diet mentality" which
keeps most people overweight.

3. How to lose weight by having a better sex
life.

4. Exercise information for those who want to
lose weight.

5. Nutritional information when you have a
weight or overeating problem.

Some of the names in this book have been
changed, but the facts are accurate.

TABLE OF CONTENTS

PART 3   LIVING THE NATURALLY THIN LIFE

PART I

THE TRUTH ABOUT DIETING

Chapter 1

WHY DIETS STILL DON'T WORK

Eight years ago when I published my first book, *DIETS DON'T WORK*, many people laughed when they heard the title. "Is this a joke book?" one asked.

Now, after doing over 700 radio, newspaper, and television interviews, after a half million Americans have read *DIETS DON'T WORK*, and after watching many celebrities who lost weight on a diet begin to gain their weight back, I say it is time for all of us to take a stand, open our windows, stick our heads out and scream to the world, "Diets still don't work!"

DIETS STILL DON'T WORK!

This book, *DIETS STILL DON'T WORK*, offers hope that everyone can be what I call a "Naturally Thin Person." Naturally thin is a natural state into which all humans are born. Naturally thin people stay thin all their lives without ever dieting or counting calories. They eat exactly what they want and never gain weight. The promise of this book is to turn you into a naturally thin person.

Despite what you have probably been told, eating too much is not a disease. It is a learned behavior, and this fact should offer you hope. It means that if you eat too much, you can change your habits. If you were able to learn how to overeat, you can also learn how to eat like a naturally thin person.

WHERE IT ALL BEGAN

Between the ages of thirty and forty, I had lost over 2,000 pounds from dieting—not all at once, of course, but on successive diets. During this period I owned twenty six health clubs in the west and southwest. I had been on a hundred different diets during that ten year period and was successful every time at reaching my weight loss goal. But my weight always returned once I stopped dieting.

Each diet had a maintenance plan to follow after I lost my weight. As I think back, the longest I ever stayed on maintenance was about three hours.

At first, ending a diet was not a problem. The weight came back very slowly over a long period of time. When I gained too much back to be comfortable, I would find and go on a new diet. 26,000 or so diets have been published since 1920, so finding a new diet was easy and, for a while, dieting worked reasonably well for me.

The problem was that every time I lost my extra 20 to 40 pounds, it was taking longer and longer to get the weight off. And, every time I gained my weight back, it came back faster and faster.

I reached the end of my rope one Monday morning when I got up and started to go to work. I had been on a weekend-long, out-of-control, non-stop eating binge, and I found that I could not button even my largest size pants.

I was terrified. Who wouldn't be? I owned a chain of health clubs, and chubby weight loss experts are not very popular. What was even worse was that I had to call in and say that I wasn't coming to work. Have you ever had to call in "fat?"

What was I to do? I considered selling all of my health clubs and opening a chain of Italian restaurants.

Then a great idea occurred to me. Like most people, I had always had a problem going back on a diet that I had been on before. The first time was fine, but I always cringed when I thought of starting out with the monotony which always seemed to set in after the first few days of a new diet. This time, however, was different. I was desperate. Why not go on the first diet I had ever been on? I had lost 11 pounds on that diet in the first seven days.

I found the diet and got started right away. I squeezed into some old sweat pants and went to the store to buy all of the diet ingredients for the next week's menu plan. On the way to the store I saw a couple of very thin joggers and decided that this time I would diet and jog at the same time. Joggers are thin, aren't they? If I jogged and dieted simultaneously, I should lose weight twice as fast.

A week later, after jogging over 20 miles and starving myself, I climbed on the scale. I had lost one pound.

I had started out this last time with 40 pounds to lose. At the rate of a pound a week, I would have only 39 more weeks of starving and jogging ahead of me. I had the overpowering feeling that I wasn't going to make it this time.

I was stumped. I knew everything about exercise, diet, and nutrition, and yet I could no longer lose weight and keep it off. I had become more and more obsessive about eating instead of less and less. I was a success in every area of my life except weight control. My overeating and extra weight seemed to invalidate everything else I had accomplished.

Chapter 2

NEW   BREAKTHROUGHS
AND OLD

How could someone who had the willpower to figure out every other problem that life had thrown at him not be able to control his weight and eating? What was I doing wrong?

Suddenly a light bulb went on. For twenty years I had been learning everything that overweight people knew about losing weight. I had been studying the wrong people. It was as if I had been studying how poor people try to get rich. If you want to get rich and stay rich, you don't study poor people. Even if you were only a little bit smart, you would study rich people who had become rich and stayed rich.

I decided that I would begin to study naturally thin people. This idea had not occurred to me before because I had thought that all naturally thin people stayed thin because their bodies burned food faster than other people's bodies. I was convinced that it was their high metabolism rate which should be given credit.

But...what if the answer were something else? What if they knew something that I did not know? Something that I may have forgotten. After all, I too had been a naturally thin person up until age thirty.

At first I talked to the thin people who had at one time been fat. I limited this group to those who had kept their weight off for at least five years.

Any weight loss organization that is worth its salt knows the statistics on dieting: out of every 200 people who go on any weight loss diet, approximately 190 fail. These 190 begin to gain back whatever weight they have lost before they even reach their weight loss goal.

Sounds awful doesn't it? Actually, this part of the statistic turns out to be the good news. The worst part is that 9 of the 10 who make it to their goal gain their weight back within 5 years.

Depressing, isn't it? Using diets, your chances of losing your weight and keeping it off for at least 5 years is only 1 in 200. If you like those odds, the casinos in Las Vegas are going to love to meet you.

Studying thin people who had lost their weight and kept it off by dieting—that 1/2 of 1 percent of dieters—proved to be a dead end. These "Artificially Thin People," as I began to call them, seemed to have compulsive personalities. They used to overeat compulsively—now they diet, count calories, worry about gaining their weight back, and undereat compulsively. I felt like I was around someone who was holding a beach ball under the water while they went through life. They spent all of their energy, time, and attention on what they ate or what they didn't eat...on how much they gained or how much they lost...on how much they had exercised or in worrying that they hadn't done enough. Their compulsive behavior drove people around them crazy and was not the way I wanted to live the rest of my life.

THE REALLY BAD NEWS

One day as I was looking through the monthly weight and measurement files in my health club, I ran across an old record of one of my members who had been around dieting and exercising for 20 years. As I compared her present day records with those 20 year old ones, I discovered something shocking. Her present day weight and measurements were bigger than when she had first started dieting and exercising. An idea began to form in my head.

Some people go to a health club to gain weight. What would happen if I were to put underweight people on the same diet that overweight people went on to lose weight?

I offered a special experimental weight gaining program to anyone who wanted to participate. My skinny members were very anxious to try out this new program.

If you have ever been underweight, you know that it is very hard to gain weight. You can stuff yourself with extra calories and exercise until you drop and you may only gain a few pounds which will quickly disappear as soon as you stop exercising and eating.

If you are overweight, you may not feel very sorry for these individuals, but these folks are a lot like you. Many times they also feel that their bodies are "ugly" and they, too, try to camouflage their faults with clothing. Most of the time they are too embarrassed to put on a bathing suit and go to the beach, and they often become withdrawn and miserable.

My "Special Weight Gain Program" was a hit. I told each person that they would be given a special eating program which they were to follow exactly for three days. I also warned them that they would probably feel some side effects from the program. Some of them might feel hungry, irritable, cranky, or tired, and they would probably start to want to eat things which were not on their eating program.

They all said that nothing mattered except gaining weight and they would promise to follow the eating program exactly.

After the first day, participants came in, usually complaining about how bad they felt: headaches, weakness, inability to concentrate. "Good!" I would say. "That means the program is working."

The second and third days they would stagger in and say, "I really feel rotten today! It must REALLY be working, huh?"

These skinny people had never been on a weight loss diet before and did not realize that they were on the very same popular, well balanced, weight loss diets that we have all been on.

On the fourth day we allowed them to get on the scale for the first time since the diet had started. Guess what happened?

Yes. They had lost weight. The average weight loss was 3 to 7 pounds. This weight loss turned out to be a surprise to them, and most of them were irate. They jumped up and down and complained that I must have made a mistake. They wanted to GAIN weight, not LOSE weight!

Eventually I calmed them down by letting them know that, on this program, what had happened was exactly what was supposed to happen. Now they were to stop the diet and simply return to eating the way they had before the diet started.

They were very disillusioned by this time, but since they were going to return to normal eating anyway, they easily agreed.

What happened? The same thing that happens to overweight people. They very quickly not only gained back the weight they had lost, but also put on a couple of extra pounds.

The skinny people were thrilled. For the first time in their lives, they had been able to gain weight in a short period of time. When their weight gain leveled off, they would come back to me and beg to be given back their diet so that they could gain some more weight.

I would give them the same diet for the same three day period and guess what happened? Yes, they lost weight. But strangely enough, not as much as the time before. The average weight losses the second time were only 1 to 5 pounds even though the diet was followed exactly the same way and for the same amount of time.

"Don't worry," I would say. "Just go off the diet and eat normally."

They would follow these instructions and would gain whatever they had lost plus a few pounds more.

I kept putting them on the diet and taking them off until they had gained all of the weight they wanted. Most of them got to the point that they would not lose anything while on the diet, but would begin to gain weight again as soon as the diet stopped.

11

Do you see any humor in this? Does it sound like the story of your life?

You see, I was wrong when I said diets don't work. Diets DO work! They work in reverse. They make most people gain weight in the long run. Ask the people you know who have dieted over a long period of their lives if they don't weigh more today than the day that they went on their very first diet. Most will say yes.

WHY?

Why does this happen? I've discovered two very basic reasons. One is that diets lower your metabolism (the rate that your body burns food). When the amount of food that your body has been receiving drops drastically, your body figures that the planet has temporarily run out of food and your metabolism slows down in order to compensate. The problem is that when you go back to normal eating, your metabolism does not seem to pop right back up to where it started. It moves up very cautiously. Some people have dieted so often that they can actually starve and not lose any weight at all.

The other reason why diets don't work, however, seems to be the most important. I have discovered that ANYTHING THAT HUMAN BEINGS ARE DEPRIVED OF, THEY BECOME OB- SESSIVE ABOUT.

Diets are supposed to have you think less about food, but just the reverse happens. We begin to think about food all of the time. We even have dreams about eating.

Right after *DIETS DON'T WORK* was first published, I began to receive countless letters from readers who were thrilled that they were losing weight without dieting. They were most grateful, however, because they had finally lost their obsession about food. They were amazed that this long time problem had vanished.

IF YOU WANT TO BE NATURALLY THIN...STUDY NATURALLY THIN PEOPLE

Around this same time I started studying people who had never had a weight problem. I was right that some of them had high metabolisms. They ate a lot and their bodies burned their intake efficiently. Most of them were young. I knew, that like me, their bodies would eventually slow down and they would have the same problem I experienced. Some of the naturally thin people, however, gave me a glimmer of hope. Even as they grew older and their metabolisms slowed down, their eating slowed down. How did they do it?

I would ask these naturally thin people questions that every fat person knows the answers to, such as, "How many calories are in (whatever food they were eating)?" To my amazement, they had no clue. After repeating this type of questioning with many of these naturally thin people and getting the same response, I saw the light. Only fat people knew about calories.

Somehow the naturally thin people avoided putting more food in their bodies than needed by some magic which they did not seem able to explain.

If I could just figure out how they avoided overeating without dieting or depriving themselves of whatever they wanted, I would have the secret to losing weight and keeping it off.

These naturally thin people, however, had different eating habits. Some ate well balanced meals while others ate mostly fast foods. Some exercised regularly, but some did not exercise at all. Some ate three meals a day, some ate one, and some ate six times a day.

I knew that I was on the right track and that there was an answer to losing weight and keeping it off without effort or struggle. Soon I was to discover what that answer was.

THE SECRET OF
NATURALLY THIN PEOPLE

I found out what the naturally thin person's secrets were and they amazed me by their simplicity. These are some of the things I learned.

*For almost everyone, being thin is a natural state.

*It can be as easy and as natural to lose weight as it is to gain it.

*Naturally thin people do four simple things that fat people don't, and they never diet.

*People gain and keep weight for specific reasons and there are specific ways to get and keep weight off.

*You can become and stay thin naturally without effort or struggle and enjoy yourself in the process.

What I discovered wasn't just another list of do's and don't's. It was a way of thinking about food and about eating based on a simple, natural principle. If you begin to practice that principle, this new way of thinking, feeling, and behaving, then you're on the verge of having your naturally thin body back.

It's not weight that's the real problem—it's the mentality behind it. Get rid of the mentality, and the weight comes off by itself, as quickly and as naturally as it was put on.

I know because I lost my weight and keep it off without dieting. So did thousands of people

I shared the process with in my Diets Don't Work Weekend Workshops, and hundreds of thousands of people who read and used the information from *DIETS DON'T WORK*. So did a special lady named Leah, who has kept the 40 pounds she lost from *DIETS DON'T WORK* off for the last eleven years and whom I fell in love with and married.

We began to think like naturally thin people, feel like naturally thin people, and behave like naturally thin people. We eat real food, not diet food. We now know that if we want ice cream, a thousand carrot sticks won't satisfy us.

We don't have to think about our weight anymore. We feel happier, freer, healthier, and more energetic than we ever have in our lives. There's a joy and rightness about living now, as if we discovered some fountain of youth that was there all along. And what we learned about weight has affected every other area of our lives.

This book deals with more than just taking off pounds. It offers a way of living which will give you joy and peace as you take off pounds. My goal in writing this book is to END WEIGHT AS A PROBLEM IN YOUR LIFE FOREVER, so that you can go on to do all those things you were going to do AFTER you lost your weight. Use the following exercise to begin to discover what your life will be like as a naturally thin person.

EXERCISE (2 minutes)

If you woke up tomorrow morning with a new naturally thin body and were exactly the weight you wanted to be, what three things would you do? If you need more room to write out your answers, use additional paper and staple it to this page.

a.

b.

c.

As you think of more things to do after you become naturally thin, add to this list. As you read through the book, refer back to this list and begin to act like a naturally thin person by doing the things on your list, one at a time—easiest things first.

The bottom line of *DIETS STILL DON'T WORK* is . . . If you want to be rich, don't study poor people or do what poor people do. Study and do what rich people do if you want to become and stay rich.

If you want to be naturally thin, don't study or do what fat dieters do. Study and do what naturally thin people do. These naturally thin people have the answers.

DIETS DON'T WORK and *DIETS STILL DON'T WORK* are both about becoming and staying "naturally thin." If this possibility intrigues you, read on.

Chapter 3

ENDING WEIGHT AND OVEREATING DISORDERS AS A PROBLEM FOR EVERYONE BY 2000 A.D.

Wouldn't the world be a better place for everyone if that same thought and energy that is thrown away on dieting could be used to make a difference in the world? What a waste! Intelligent, talented, wonderful people are spending enormous amounts of time dieting and beating themselves up about their weight and eating.

What would it take to end weight and overeating as a problem for everyone by 2000 A.D.? First, it will take ending weight and overeating as a problem for you. You do make a difference. Without you, the vision of the end of weight problems and overeating is not possible.

DIETS STILL DON'T WORK and *DIETS DON'T WORK* are about fitting your weight and eating goals into your life and learning to deal with them successfully rather than having weight and overeating be what your life is about.

You may be one of the many who have failed over and over again at putting an end to your weight and eating problems, but you were probably operating on old information. You kept using the same old diet information to decide what action to take. You may have been surprised each time that you didn't get very far with your weight loss program or if you did, you gained back whatever you had lost plus a few pounds more.

No wonder! You kept doing the same thing over and over again, hoping for a different result and blaming yourself if you failed. That is crazy!

What I am asking you to do is very difficult. I want you to pretend to forget everything you know or think you know about losing weight.

Nothing is wrong with you. Trust whatever path you have chosen to handle your weight and eating. The journey you have selected may be longer than someone next to you, but so what? You are resolving the source of overeating and dissatisfaction in your life. Maybe you have more to deal with than someone else. Your past life may have been more complicated.

Let's tackle losing weight, one step at a time. First things first.

WHERE ARE YOU, RIGHT NOW?

The following exercises will help you gain the specific insights that you'll need to become a naturally thin person. Whatever you do, don't use any of the information you gather as a club to beat yourself up with. Your purpose is simply to tell the truth about where you are now and how you feel about yourself. Please take the time to write down the answers to the exercises carefully and experience what you feel as you are doing them.

EXERCISE (3 minutes)

1. "My present weight in the morning is: _____. I wear size _____ pants and size _____ dress or coat. My measurements are: _____ (waist), _____ (abdomen), _____ (upper part of right arm), _____ (upper part of right thigh)."

This is your starting place. From time to time you will probably want to come back to this page in order to acknowledge how far you have come.

MAKING IT YOURS

This book has been carefully designed to let you produce specific and measurable results. It is intended to give you the experience of being a naturally thin person that people get in my Diets Don't Work Weekend Workshops. It is your personal workbook, a private diary that is yours and yours alone.

The exercises in each chapter are for your eyes only, unless you choose otherwise. They were designed as a way for you to discover: 1) how the unwanted pounds got on your body in the first place, 2) what has been in the way of taking your weight off and keeping it off, and 3) what it will take for you to become a naturally thin person once and for all.

Everyone who reads this book will discover different personal insights. Having these insights will allow you to see how you gained your weight and why it stays. In other words, reading this book will help you find out what really causes you to overeat and what to do about it. You'll be in a position to choose for yourself whether you want to live and eat like a fat person or like a naturally thin person. You've never really been in a position to make that choice before because of what I call the "Diet Mentality."

22

The Diet Mentality, a way of thinking in regard to losing weight and eating, sets up rules and regulations for losing weight and eating. Like a pair of colored glasses, your Diet Mentality colors whatever you see. The Diet Mentality twists your thinking so that even when you try to follow the rules, you still wind up failing. Not only do you fail, but you blame yourself, not the diet for your failure.

DIETS STILL DON'T WORK will give you an alternate way of thinking in regard to losing weight and eating. *DIETS STILL DON'T WORK* contains a new set of rules and regulations which you probably have never considered, a way to be successful even if you have failed in the past. By working through the following exercises, you will know how to be a naturally thin person by the time you get to the end of this book.

BEGINNING TO BE
YOUR OWN BEST FRIEND

One of the most devastating things about the mental condition that I named the Diet Mentality is that it encourages you to hate yourself and your body and to treat yourself accordingly. The *DIETS STILL DON'T WORK* approach to the whole issue of weight loss is to be kind, positive, and gentle with yourself. Being overweight is not a crime. The person inside your body, the

23

real you, is a capable and worthy individual, even if you presently don't think so.

I invite you to put self-recrimination aside while you read this book and start now to see what it would be like to be loving toward yourself. We're all indoctrinated with the idea that we have to use harsh discipline on ourselves to get results. In fact, in the long run just the opposite is true.

There are probably hundreds of ways that you daily deprive yourself or treat yourself like a second–class person. In the next exercise you get to play the part of your best friend, someone who knows everything about you. You're going to make lists of all the things that, if someone did them for you, would make you feel cared about and appreciated. This is an extremely important exercise. The purpose of it right now is for you to get down in black and white all of the many ways in which you are not now treating yourself like a naturally thin person.

I've divided the list into five categories with space for five items under each category.

EXERCISES (15 minutes)

1. "These are five personal things I would like to do for myself that would make me feel cared about:"

a.

b.

c.

d.

e.

2. "These are five things I would like to do for myself at work that would make me feel cared about:"
a.

b.

c.

d.

e.

3. "These are five things I would like to do around the house that would make me feel cared about:"
a.

b.

c.

d.

e.

4. "These are five things I would like to do in my relationships that would make me feel cared about:"

a.

b.

c.

d.

e.

5. "These are five things I would like to do or have done for my body that would make me feel cared about:"

a.

b.

c.

d.

e.

Thank you for taking the time and energy to write out your answers. Over the last eight years I have met thousands of people who read *DIETS DON'T WORK*. Every one of those who had lost all of their weight and kept it off had WRITTEN OUT THE ANSWERS TO THE QUESTIONS IN THEIR BOOKS. Those who were still struggling with their weight may have thought about the answers but did not take the time to write them down. Writing the answers down creates results for the reader that just thinking about the answers does not. I know how difficult it is to write in a book after having been told for years in school not to. Your answers in this book will prove not only to be a logical place to keep this information, but you will also have the answers when you go back and review this information days or years from now. Do not think too much when you answer the questions. If you get stuck, just keep writing. Make something up. You will discover when you go back and read over what you have written that some of your made up answers may begin to make a lot of sense. Lighten up. This is not a test.

If you are reading the book with someone such as your husband, wife, daughter or son, you may use the same book if you want to, but use a different color of ink to keep your answers separate. Doing the book together is a great way to find out things about each other. You will also learn how to support each other in being naturally thin.

If you need more room than is provided, use additional paper and staple it to the page you are using. Hopefully I have provided enough space for your answers, but if not, do not let the limited space limit your writing.

Part II:

HOW TO DISMANTLE THE DIET MENTALITY

Chapter 4

REASONS WHY YOU
STILL OVEREAT

EATING TRIGGERS

What is a "trigger?" In dealing with behavioral terminology, a trigger is when something happens or someone does something and you suddenly have an automatic reaction. The behavior that shows up in you is sometimes not the smartest way to react and you can end up damaging yourself or someone else.

"TRIGGER EATING" is the term I use to describe automatic eating. For most people, it is impossible to control, as if you become unconscious and wake up after what seems like a bad dream of overeating. You don't usually remember the exact moment you became unconscious, and the only time you realize that you were unconscious is when you wake up from this frenzy of overeating.

If you are seized with "TRIGGER EATING," it is essential NOT to beat yourself up. The best thing you can do is to look to see exactly what set you off and find an alternative to impulsive eating.

You may need to save the next group of questions until your next bout of "TRIGGER EATING."

Look over the following questions and write down however much of the information you can recall at this time.

THE LAST TIME YOU WERE TRIGGERED:

EXERCISE (8 minutes)

What were the exact words that were said by the person or persons that triggered you or what was the exact event that triggered you before you overate? Be as precise as possible. Describe exactly what happened and what was said:

What were the exact words that were said by you or what were the thoughts you were having during the time you were triggered? Describe step by step exactly what you did.:

What do you suppose you could do to desensitize those words, thoughts, or events that trigger you into being upset and overeating? Make something up if you have to. Don't think. Just write down any solution that occurs to you from start to finish no matter how unreasonable it may seem.:

Thank you for writing out your answers. Now go back and read over what you wrote. As you read your answers, see if you can imagine the same circumstance happening again and try to picture yourself responding in some other way which would be more appropriate than eating.

Did you succeed? _____
Today's date: _____

If you are not convinced that you will be able to react like a naturally thin person the next time the above circumstance happens, fold down the edge of this page. Later on, come back to this part. Read over your answers to the above questions and again imagine yourself reacting like a naturally thin person. Keep repeating this exercise until you are able to do so successfully. At that time, scratch through your above "no" answer and write "yes" as well as change the date to that on which you succeeded.

THE BIG TWELVE

In *DIETS DON'T WORK* I laid out thirty typical reasons for overeating that the people in my weekend workshops usually came up with. Over the last eight years I have found that the main reasons most people overeat fall into the following twelve categories.

1. UNCONSCIOUS EATING (EATING WITHOUT THINKING)

2. FEELING STRESS OR TENSION

3. NOT GETTING WHAT YOU WANT

4. RESISTING DOING SOMETHING THAT YOU DON'T WANT TO DO

5. WITHHOLDING THOUGHTS, FEELINGS, OR INFORMATION

6. BEING BORED

7. SEEKING PLEASURE

8. SCARCITY EATING

9. TUMESCENCE (PENT UP SEXUAL ENERGY)

10. SEEKING APPROVAL

11. TO AVOID FEELINGS

12. FEELING EMOTIONALLY EMPTY

Which of these reasons do you use (or should I say, "Uses you?") to overeat? Please "write" out specific situations or times when you were affected by any of these eating triggers. Write the first thought that occurs to you. Don't edit what you write. Write as fast as you can and keep writing until your mind is a blank. If you think of something else later on, you can always come back and add to what you have already written.

1.UNCONSCIOUS EATING (EATING WITHOUT THINKING):

"These are the specific situations and times that I go unconscious and automatically overeat:"

2. FEELING STRESS OR TENSION: For many people, stress is the number one trigger for overeating.

"These are the specific situations and times that I overeat because I am feeling stress or tension:"

3. YOU ARE NOT GETTING WHAT YOU WANT: Disappointment, frustration, or failure may set into motion a need for some feeling of satisfaction. If you can't have whatever you are being denied, at least you can have as much food as you can get your hands on.

"I overeat when I don't get what I want. This is a list of what I want that I am not getting:"

4. RESISTING DOING SOMETHING THAT YOU DON'T WANT TO DO:

"I overeat when I am resisting doing the following things:"

5. WITHHOLDING THOUGHTS, FEELINGS, OR INFORMATION: What is a "withhold?" A withhold is anything that you do not disclose to someone else. We all withhold thoughts, feelings, or information. We withhold constantly and we always have a reason to withhold. Although it would not make sense to walk around and spurt out every thought, feeling, and every bit of information that we become aware of, withholds can be a big cause of unconscious overeating.

EXERCISES (15 minutes)

A. List at least five big or little thoughts, feelings, or information that you have withheld from the person closest to you:

B. List at least five big or little thoughts, feelings, or information that you have withheld from your most important relative, other than your spouse:

C. List at least five big or little thoughts, feelings, or information that you have withheld from one of your friends:

D. List at least five big or little thoughts, feelings, or information that you have withheld from someone that either has died or that you have lost touch with:

E. List at least five big or little thoughts, feelings, or information that you have withheld from your boss, someone important that works for you, or someone important in your life that could cause you a problem if you told them about your withhold:

Look back over the above withholds and see if any of them seem to be a trigger that causes you to overeat. At this point, do not attempt to do anything about the withholds. I have a solution later on in the book for the eating caused by withholds.

6. BEING BORED:
"These are the specific situations and times that I get bored and overeat:"

7. SEEKING PLEASURE:
"These are the specific situations and times that I overeat for pleasure or fun:"

8. SCARCITY EATING: (If I don't eat it now, I won't get it later.)

"These are the specific situations and times that bring up the feelings or thoughts of scarcity in me which cause me to overeat:"

9. TUMESCENCE: Pronounced "TU-MESS-ENCE" is defined in the book, *THE ONE HOUR ORGASM*, as pent up sexual energy.

THE ONE HOUR ORGASM, is based on the discoveries of Dr. W. Victor Baranco of More

University who presents courses in human sensuality in the United States and Canada.

One of Dr. Baranco's discoveries was that if sexual energy, tumescence, builds up without being relieved, it can cause a person to become agitated, irritable, highly sensitive, clumsy, anxious, on edge, cranky, hostile, hypercritical, bad tempered, and physically uncomfortable. Many times women will report feeling highly tumesced just prior to their menstrual and ovulation cycles. Dr. Baranco found that men, although they do not have menstrual or ovulation cycles, become tumesced when they are around anyone who is tumesced.

Cravings for certain types of food are common at times of high tumescence. Eating chocolate, fried foods, pastries, or other heavy, greasy foods with high levels of oil or fat was found to bring down tumescent levels from uncomfortable physical and emotional highs to comfortable levels. The side effect, however, of eating heavy, greasy food is usually weight gain and lack of ability to lose weight.

(Complete information about solutions for pleasurably reducing tumescence without overeating can be found in the book *THE ONE HOUR ORGASM*. See last page of this book for details.)

"These are the specific signs and times that I overeat because I am tumesced:"

10. SEEKING APPROVAI : To make someone happy.

"These are the specific people that I attempt to make happy by overeating and the situations and times that I overeat around them:"

A twenty two year old woman named Melva from Houston, said: "My Father was always cooking for me and offering me food. It made him happy when I ate his wonderful cooking. One day I realized that every time I ate to make him happy, I was making myself unhappy by getting fat. We had a talk. He didn't realize how unhappy I was, being overweight. We made a deal that he would not offer food unless I first asked for it. I am at my ideal weight now, and he is so proud of me."

11. TO AVOID FEELINGS:
These are the specific feelings that I try to avoid feeling by eatin·"

12. FEELING EMPTY:
"I overeat, although I am not hungry, because I am feeling empty for the following reasons:"

Thank you for writing out your answers. Later on in our journey to the naturally thin you, we will look for naturally thin solutions to these issues.

CAN YOU NAME THAT TUNE?

At this time, go back over your answers and see if you can give a name to a particular type of eating that you do. For example, under "Pleasure eating" you may describe a particular behavior that you find yourself exhibiting when on vacation. You feel obliged to savor local delicacies because they usually are not available to you at home. You may decide to label this as "Souvenir eating."

Another favorite type of eating could be when you feel a vague craving to eat something, but you cannot figure out exactly what it is that you want. A good label for this might be "Grazing," since you usually behave by starting at one end of the kitchen or refrigerator and slowly eating your way to the other end in order to find what you are looking for. A name you could give to a bout of nonstop eating would be something like "Feeding Frenzy." Make up labels or names which will be easy for you to remember and list them below

At this point you may be feeling depressed or giddy. Don't worry. Everything is going to turn out all right.

This may be your first time down this path to a naturally thin life, but I have been down it thousands of times with thousands of people and I know something that you don't know. Everything is going to turn out and you are going to be just fine.

EXERCISES (10 minutes)

1. Go back to the beginning of your weight problem. What happened in your life just before you began to gain weight? How old were you? What was happening in your relationships? What was your money situation? How successful did you consider yourself at the time? Was there some crisis, upset, trauma, or pressure in your life at that time? Write out as much detail as possible

2. What decisions did you make during the above times in regard to eating?

Thank you for writing whatever you recalled during the above exercise. If any more information occurs to you, please return to this section and add to your answers.

Chapter 5

WHY YOU STILL CAN'T GET
THERE FROM HERE

One of the reasons you may be feeling a little hopeless right now is that you are being directed down an unfamiliar trail. The voices in your head may be screaming things such as "When are we going to get started? I want to lose weight, not answer questions! Where's the beef?"

IMPATIENCE...A CURSE

One of the biggest traps when a person is on the way to having a naturally thin body and behavior is being in a hurry. Trying to go too fast is almost always destructive. "Speeding," the term I give to this kind of behavior, does not work.

THE VICIOUS CYCLE
OF BEING IMPATIENT

Put a check mark by the following items that reflect the cycle of what happens when you get in a hurry to lose weight:
- "I get in a hurry.
- I start doing what fat people do, not what naturally thin do.
- I begin to feel bad about myself and start beating myself up.
- I start overeating.
- I feel worse about myself and beat myself up even more.
- I either give up or get in a bigger hurry to lose weight and take drastic actions.
- I fail and start overeating again."

As you can imagine, the above scenario is a no win situation. In your journey to being a naturally thin person for the rest of your life, speeding should be a signal to you that you need to slow down. Breathe. Smell the flowers. Lighten up. If you need to, go beat a pillow and scream until you can't lift your arms or go for a long walk and don't start back until you are ready to practice being naturally thin again.

IT LOOKS HOPELESS

What is the best way to predict how you are going to behave and perform in the future? Look at how you behaved and performed in the past. Look at your record, your history. We change very little unless something drastic happens.

Approximately how many times have you decided to lose weight?

How many times have you lost weight only to gain it back again?

List the diets and exercise programs you have started:

With all of your reasons why you want to lose your weight and keep it off permanently, why do you imagine you are still struggling with the problem?

54

How many times have you promised that you were going to do something that would support you in losing weight or not overeating and broken your promise?

Your promises may be worth a lot in every other area of your life, but they seem to be worthless in this one. If commitment is measured by the consistent results you produce, you seem to be committed to staying overweight and to overeating. No matter what you have said, done, or promised...here you are.

You may be feeling very beat up about now, but instead of feeling bad, why not be curious? How could it be that a person who is trustworthy in many other areas of life cannot be trusted around food or eating? Why is it that you eventually break every promise that you make in the area of eating and weight? Do you suddenly get brain damage when you get near food?

If you weren't so close to the situation and were an objective scientist, you would suspect that something else is the real problem. Maybe you keep going down the wrong path and that is why you keep winding up in the wrong place.

Chapter 6

HOW THIN PEOPLE
THINK AND EAT

THE SECRET

Are you ready for the big secret? Are you
ready to find out how naturally thin people can
eat exactly what they want without gaining
weight? It's going to sound deceptively simple,
but don't be fooled. It's the simplest and yet may
be the most difficult challenge you've ever faced.

What makes eating like a naturally thin person
difficult is that some basic, fundamental shifts in
how you now approach food, eating, yourself,
and your life are involved. As you read, imagine
yourself behind that naturally thin person's eyes
and notice how you feel.

In studying naturally thin people, I learned that they do four fundamental things when they eat that fat people don't.

1. They don't eat unless their body is HUNGRY.

2. They eat EXACTLY what they want—EXACTLY what will satisfy them.

3. They don't eat unconsciously; they ENJOY every bite of what they are eating and they are aware of the effect the food is having on their bodies.

4. They stop eating when their bodies are no longer hungry.

Is their secret as simple as that? I couldn't believe that this was the secret and tried to make it more complicated. The secret had to be the kind of food they ate or their metabolisms. But I found that some naturally thin people had low metabolisms and some had high metabolisms. Some eat junk food, and some eat health food. Some eat an early dinner, and some eat late at night. Some eat quickly, others eat slowly. The only habits they all have in common are that they eat only when their bodies get HUNGRY, they eat EXACTLY what will satisfy them, they ENJOY and are aware of every bite they take and of the effect the food is having on their bodies, and they stop when their bodies are NO LONGER HUNGRY.

IF YOU STOP AND THINK ABOUT IT, THAT'S HOW CHILDREN AND ANIMALS EAT. THE WAY THAT NATURALLY THIN PEOPLE EAT IS THE NATURAL APPROACH TO EATING.

Let's take those four eating characteristics one at a time and examine some possible pitfalls.

1. NATURALLY THIN PEOPLE EAT ONLY BECAUSE THEY'RE HUNGRY. Naturally thin people don't eat because they don't want to do something or because they are feeling anxious, as fat people often do. Their days don't revolve around food. Sometimes they say, "Oh, I forgot to eat today." The only time overeaters forget to eat is when they are asleep or unconscious, but if naturally thin people aren't hungry, they don't think about food. It isn't an issue in their lives, since they give themselves permission to eat exactly what they want.

It wouldn't occur to them to eat for any of the reasons we do—they eat only because their bodies are hungry. They don't waste food by eating more than their bodies need. Food is just food, not love, comfort, sex, or companionship.

2. NATURALLY THIN PEOPLE EAT EXACTLY WHAT THEY WANT—EXACTLY WHAT WILL

SATISFY THEM. Naturally thin people do a funny thing before they sit down to a meal, they usually take the time to ask themselves what they want to eat. Not to eat exactly what is satisfying would be a foreign concept to them. They look to see what they want before they start eating.

They don't ask themselves what they shouldn't eat; they ask themselves what they want to eat. They seem to have some sort of inner barometer that tells them not only what would taste good at that particular moment, but also what would satisfy their bodies' wants and needs.

They know that if they want a steak, a head of lettuce isn't going to satisfy them. If they really want a baked potato, cottage cheese isn't going to make them happy. If they want chocolate ice cream, even a thousand carrot sticks aren't going to satisfy their craving!

Normally, naturally thin people are finicky eaters—they don't eat what they don't want. They don't eat just to be eating; they eat because a particular food rings a loud bell for them and because they are hungry.

If they're out to lunch and nothing on the menu sounds tantalizing, either they'll leave and go elsewhere, or they'll order a token serving just to take the edge off their hunger. They do strange things, like not finishing everything on their plates. If a plate containing meat, vegetables, and potatoes is set in front of them, they'll only eat what they like. They may eat just the meat and the spinach, for example, and leave behind a mound of mashed potatoes. Or they may not touch the meat and eat a big dessert instead. Sometimes, if they have the option, they may not eat at all. They'll do something else instead. THEY KNOW THERE WILL ALWAYS BE ANOTHER MEAL.

And there's one thing naturally thin people never do—they never go on a diet. ONLY FAT PEOPLE DIET!

3. NATURALLY THIN PEOPLE EAT CONSCIOUSLY AND ENJOY EVERY BITE. They are conscious of what they're eating and the effect the food is having on their bodies. SINCE THEY PAY ATTENTION AND ENJOY EVERY BITE OF WHAT THEY'RE EATING, THEY'RE SATISFIED WITH LESS AND ENJOY THEIR FOOD MORE!

Overeaters never get tired of eating because they eat while thinking about everything except the food on their plates, and they seldom even taste their food until the end of the meal.

Because naturally thin people are aware and conscious when they're eating, they know when their body reaches the "not hungry level." Most fat people have no idea how hungry they are before, while, or after they eat. Naturally thin people keep tuned in to their bodies, and they know when their bodies aren't hungry anymore.

Many naturally thin people are ignorant about food. They don't know anything about diets, and the process of counting calories baffles them. They only know four things: when they're hungry, exactly what they want to eat, that they are going to enjoy each bite of food they put in their mouths or not eat it, and when their bodies are no longer hungry. When you think about it, those points are all you really need to know in order to begin to lose weight and to transform your Diet Mentality into a Naturally Thin Mentality.

4. NATURALLY THIN PEOPLE STOP EATING WHEN THEIR BODIES ARE NO LONGER HUNGRY. Did you ever have someone try to press more food on you? Naturally thin people have three words that stop people from trying to get them to eat more than they want. They say, "I'm not hungry," and if pressed, they just apologetically keep repeating those three words.

Haven't you seen a naturally thin person stop eating right in the middle of an expensive meal, push the plate away, and feel no guilt whatsoever? Have you ever seen them wrap up and save as little as two bites of food, or take all but two sips of a soft drink and put it back in the refrigerator? Have you ever asked them why they don't finish what they are eating or drinking, and hear them say, "I'm not hungry. I'll finish it later."? Doggie bags were invented for naturally thin people. Fat people eat everything that lands on the table.

Naturally thin people don't care whether or not they're in the Clean Plate Club. They will occasionally overeat, but they don't give occasional overeating a second thought. They treat food as if it were their servant, not their master. They don't pay a lot of attention to it. Sometimes they will ignore it, leave food sitting on their plate, and even throw it away!

Who are these people who are so ignorant they don't know the number of calories in a chocolate chip cookie, who don't even know what they do to stay thin? Why are naturally thin people like that, and how did they get that way?

The answer is that they didn't do anything and they don't know anything—that's just the point. Being thin is a natural state. We are the ones who have done something, who had added something to nature. We're the ones who have created the myths and the patterns and the rules that make and keep us fat. Take those away, and what you have is a natural state—naturally thin. The naturally thin are like animals in the wild, following their bodies' instincts from moment to moment.

It's not that thin people don't enjoy food— they do. Most of them probably enjoy it more than we do because they actually taste it. I noticed when I would buy an ice cream cone, the first bite would taste just great. After the second or third bite, I actually couldn't taste the flavor anymore—all I tasted was cold. If a naturally thin person stopped enjoying the ice cream, he would probably toss the rest of it away or save it for later.

I was amazed that naturally thin people didn't use food as a reward. They reward themselves with other things. You see, in order to be effective, a reward has to be just a little bit extravagant. Naturally thin people sometimes think it's extravagant to take off to see an afternoon movie or to spend more money than they should on some new clothes, but since food is just food to them, it is of little use to them as a reward. They can't use it as a weapon against themselves or others. To them eating is like breathing—neither good nor bad.

They don't "graze" because they always have something particular in mind when they eat. They go after a specific food, rather than food in the abstract. They don't indulge in scarcity eating because it never occurs to them that food is scarce. THERE WILL ALWAYS BE MORE. Naturally thin people believe that food is all around them, there for the taking whenever they want it, so they never feel deprived. They have permission from themselves to eat exactly what they want whenever they get hungry, so they feel no urgency.

EXERCISES (8 minutes)

1. "These are the fears I have about eating ONLY when my body is hungry:"

a.

b.

c.

d.

e.

2. "These are the fears I have about eating EXACTLY what I want:"

a.

b.

c.

d.

e.

3. "These are the fears about what would happen if I had to stay conscious and ENJOY every bite I ate:"

a.

b.

c.

d.

e.

4. "These are the things that might prevent me from stopping eating the moment my body is no longer hungry:"
   a.

   b.

   c.

   d.

   e.

Naturally thin people also assume that what their body tells them to eat is exactly what they need to stay healthy. If all they want to eat on a certain day when they get hungry is three chocolate bars, that's what they have. They may not get the chocolate craving again for a month. Because they give themselves permission to eat the chocolate when they really want it, the craving doesn't have control over them. The next day, they may only want vegetables or meat or bread. They trust their bodies' instincts, even when those instincts seem crazy.

I know one naturally thin person who is normally a vegetarian, but about every three months she gets an insatiable craving for two Big Macs, a large order of fries, and a chocolate shake. Nothing tastes good until she has that. When she feels the urge coming on, she heads straight for McDonalds.

Does a naturally thin person eat when he or she is not feeling well? They just ask themselves, "Am I hungry or not?"

Some naturally thin people actually like the feeling of being hungry. Hunger sensations last for about 20 seconds and then fade away. They return about 20 minutes later. Check it out the next time you get hungry.

Naturally thin people would never think to indulge in closet eating. They don't have anything to hide. In fact, they often do the opposite. They're actually more likely to eat when someone is watching and may even eat more in a restaurant or when they're out to dinner with other people than they do when they're at home alone. It's a mystery to people who are overweight how a naturally thin person can sit down and devour an enormous meal and stay thin. The answer is probably that they have waited a long time to eat and are very hungry. Tomorrow they might eat very little.

When naturally thin people are anxious, they're more likely to undereat than to overeat. They don't know about the trick of burying their emotions under food. They may do something else—pace back and forth, sleep more than they normally do, go for a long walk, or stare off into space—but when they're upset, food is often the farthest thing from their minds. They're too preoccupied to eat. Whatever is upsetting them has priority, and they can't even think about food.

It's not that thin people don't have problems, IT'S JUST THAT THEY DON'T MAKE THE CONNECTION BETWEEN PROBLEMS AND FOOD. Food is either neutral to them, fuel they use to keep their body functioning, or it's a friend. Naturally thin people don't feel deprived regarding food because they're not only eating exactly what they want, they're more apt to be doing the things that make them happy.

Are you beginning to get behind a naturally thin person's eyes and see his approach to eating and food? That's what's important. This *DIETS STILL DON'T WORK* process is not just about doing the four things naturally thin people do that fat people don't. It's about seeing where those four things come from and duplicating the naturally thin person's mentality and way of thinking. IF YOU DON'T CHANGE THE WAY YOU THINK, YOU PROBABLY WON'T BE ANY BETTER OFF THAN IF YOU'D GONE ON ANOTHER DIET. You'll just be left with another list of things you have to do and not do to fix the situation you've gotten yourself into.

The trick is to start thinking like a naturally thin person, feeling like a naturally thin person, and behaving like a naturally thin person. Be a naturally thin person right now. Change the self-image you've had. You may even have to pretend at first, until the new "rules" start to take hold.

What you will be doing is creating an environment in which the naturally thin person inside you feels comfortable and starts to emerge. The more you can allow that to happen, the more this new mentality and thinking will become yours. BE a naturally thin person inside, and it's only a matter of time before your body begins to reflect a naturally thin body outside.

Just as you can't try to put a naturally thin body underneath a fat head, you can't keep a fat body underneath a naturally thin head for long. The more you practice thinking like a naturally thin person, the more effortless it will be for your body to begin to look naturally thin. All you really have to do is enjoy being naturally thin. YOU DIDN'T HAVE TO DIET TO GAIN THE WEIGHT. IT'S ONLY FAIR THAT YOU SHOULDN'T HAVE TO DIET TO LOSE IT.

EXERCISES (5 minutes)

1. Lean back, close your eyes, and visualize yourself as a naturally thin person. Take yourself through one of your typical days, noticing what you would do, how you would interact with people, and how you would eat. Create the day exactly the way you want it to be. Take at least three minutes to do the exercise. When you finish, jot down some of the things that pleased you.

Fold this page down and come back and repeat the above exercise every day if you find it useful.

2. "These are the things that would be different about my life and about my relationship with myself and other people IF I allowed myself to live as a naturally thin person starting right now:"

a.

b.

c.

d.

e.

THIN FOR A DAY:
A TASTE OF THE THIN LIFE

The best way for you to learn how naturally thin people operate is to experience a day of approaching food the way they do. In my weekend workshop I actually serve participants a meal, during which we go through certain exercises to emphasize the Naturally Thin Mentality. I would like you to choose a day of relative freedom, say a Saturday or a Sunday, and create the experience of eating meals the way a naturally thin person would and spend the day in the Naturally Thin Mentality.

In order to actually experience the Naturally Thin Mentality, you will need to know several things. I will explore each of these matters in more detail later in the book, but for the purposes of this exercise, a brief introduction to naturally thin eating is all that is necessary.

1. RATING YOUR HUNGER. Since most people who eat too much don't have a very clear idea of what it feels like to be really hungry, I've devised a hunger scale, with 1 at the bottom and 10 at the top. One is when you're so hungry you feel faint. Ten is when you're so stuffed you can hardly move. In the middle, at 5 on the scale— which we will call "NOT HUNGRY", is the point at which your body has had enough to eat. Everything up to 4.99 is "hungry"; everything from 5.01 on up is "overeating," or "too much," what fat people call "full."

2. DISCONNECTING THE EATING MACHINE. In order to follow the third principle of naturally thin eating, that is, enjoying the eating of every bite consciously, you have to know how to get yourself off automatic. I call the process "disconnecting the eating machine." The object is to keep your attention on the food that's already in your mouth so you actually taste and enjoy it. To achieve this I have the people in my workshops put their forks down BEFORE they start to chew. Then I have them completely chew the bites that are in their mouths, squeezing out all the flavor and goodness possible before swallowing it. Only then do they pick up their forks again.

3. SIZING UP YOUR STOMACH. Before we begin the meal at the workshop, I have everyone

make a fist with their right hand. This is the approximate size of your stomach. If you're completely empty, the approximate volume of food you need to eat to satisfy your body's hunger might only fill a container about the size of your fist. How many bites of food do you suppose that would be?

4. RATING FOOD. Another thing that is useful to know before spending the day as a naturally thin eater is how to rate food. Naturally thin people generally only eat foods they really love. So I've developed a food-rating scale, again from 1 to 10, with the numbers on the bottom of the scale representing your least-favorite foods and those at the top of the scale your favorite foods of all time. Foods at the level of 1 or 2 probably have no business being in your mouth. Naturally thin people generally only eat foods that are 7s, 8s, 9s or 10s for them. This is entirely a matter of taste; everybody has different preferences. Take a few minutes and write the name of some food which would fit in these categories for you.

10 Wonderful, "Orgasmic":

9

8 Pretty Good:

7

6   OK, but Not Quality:

5

4   Not Good:

3

2   UGH!:

1

5. GETTING IN THE MOOD. Since you don't have the advantage of being in my workshop room where every aspect of your meal is controlled, you will need to know some things about how to approach eating on your naturally thin day. The first thing is to treat yourself like a naturally thin person for that whole day. When you sit down to eat your meals, pretend you're an honored guest and someone has gone to a great deal of trouble to prepare delicious food for you to eat. In the workshop we dim the lights in the room and play soft, relaxing music.

Since this will be your first day to eat like a naturally thin person, the meals you eat this day will probably be some of the most special meals you'll ever eat. If possible, you may want to eat them alone, so you can concentrate on the process of eating like a naturally thin person without any distractions. If you do eat with someone, make sure that person is participating with you, supporting you in doing the exercise.

6. DOING WHAT NATURALLY THIN PEOPLE DO WHEN THEY'RE NOT EATING.

Make out a list of at least twenty things you would really like to do or complete during your first naturally thin day. If you had one whole day to do anything that you wanted, what would you do? Maybe something is bothering you because it is not finished, such as cleaning out and organizing your refrigerator or calling people with whom you have not talked in a long time. No matter what you choose to do on your naturally thin day, just make sure that it is going to be fun or it is going to make you feel good.

Don't make the projects too complicated. Break them down into easy to do steps so that you can have the feeling of winning at each step. For instance, the first step in cleaning out your refrigerator may be to get a sponge or paper towels and cleaning solution together. Check that off as a completion. Next, take everything out of the refrigerator throwing away what you no longer want living in your refrigerator (keep only 7s, 8s, 9s and 10s). Next, clean the inside and put everything back in a place which will be its HOME until you are ready for it. The most important thing to remember is to MAKE SURE YOU FEEL LIKE YOU WIN WITH EACH ITEM THAT YOU COMPLETE, AND EITHER MAKE WHAT YOU ARE DOING FUN OR HAVE THE

ACCOMPLISHMENT MAKE YOU FEEL GOOD
THAT YOU COMPLETED IT.

If you really want to make it fun, get someone
to help you. You could get someone to read
DIETS STILL DON'T WORK along with you and
trade off helping each other to complete some of
the items that neither of you want to face alone.

Don't worry if you don't come close to com-
pleting all twenty of your items. That is not the
object of this exercise. Don't even think about
getting on your own case if you only get around
to doing a few of them. The point is to pretend
to do the things a naturally thin person might do
rather than think about food or weight and to
have fun. Write out twenty things below that you
want to do on your naturally thin day. Have fun
writing your list. Just make them up. If you
could accomplish anything that you wanted on
your naturally thin day, what would that be?

7. WHAT TO EAT? In DIETS DON'T WORK, I included the same menu that we use in the weekend workshop, but this time I want you to make up your own list of foods to eat for your naturally thin day. The only guidelines that I want you to follow on your naturally thin day are to avoid alcohol and don't eat or drink anything except water between meals.

In order to make the exercise a success, choose and make a list of a large variety of foods.

* Include and list below items you would rank as 7s, 8s, 9s or 10s, as well as "healthy" items for contrast that might be 3s or 4s.

* Include and list below a variety of fresh foods you might include such as raw fruit and vegetables.

In this next space, pre-plan exactly what you think you would like to eat and drink during each meal. Remember, you will be sampling a lot of different foods to see what they taste like when eaten by a naturally thin person. The most important part is to taste everything, but at the same time strive to eat exactly what is going to satisfy you. Try to have at least six or more items to sample at each meal. You may keep the quantities relatively small...even a bite or two of some foods may be sufficient.

Breakfast: (Meal #1)

Lunch: (Meal #2)

Dinner: (Meal #3)

Before each meal, read through the following procedure, and follow it step by step.

PROCEDURE:

1. Wait until you are hungry before you eat each meal. You may not get hungry three times a day, so you may eat less than three meals. It does not make any difference if you eat breakfast food at lunch or dinner food for breakfast. Eat exactly what you want.

2. Before each meal check your level of hunger, and write down what you think it is:

Breakfast

Lunch

Dinner

To do this, put your hands over your stomach and guess what level between 1 (starving) and 5 (your body isn't hungry) you're experiencing.

3. Before each meal, set the table and prepare your plate as if you were serving a very special person. Use your favorite china and silverware. If you like, set out flowers and candles. Turn on soft music.

4. Sit down and get ready to eat.

a. Before you start, pick up your plate and look at each item as if you had never seen it before. Pretend the food on your plate came from another planet, even though it might look like something you've eaten before.

b. Next, smell each item. Can you determine from the smell what it might taste like? If you couldn't see the food, what color does it smell like it would be?

c. Look at each morsel of food on your plate with gratitude and respect. Each food there was a living entity just a short while ago and gave up its life for your pleasure.

5. Start by picking up the most delicious item on your plate with your fingers or your fork, raise it slowly to your nose, and smell the aroma. Next, closely examine what it looks like. Describe out loud or to yourself exactly what you see and what each characteristic reminds you of. Now put the food into your mouth, but before you begin to chew, disconnect the eating machine. Put your fork down on the plate.

6. Before starting to chew, gently suck on this morsel of food for a moment. Move it around in your mouth. See if you notice different flavors when moving it to different parts of your mouth.

7. Now bite down on the food. Notice the sound it makes as you bite through it and chew it. Continue to chew the bite very slowly, and concentrate on enjoying every time your teeth cut through the food.

8. After you've chewed on this bite as much as possible and have swallowed it, notice the taste it leaves in your mouth. Savor the pleasure you can get out of the aftertaste.

9. Now go around the plate, eating one bite of each food on the plate in the same manner as you did the first. Select each bite in the order that you would rate them from most favorite to least favorite. Notice if you change your mind about their rating after you've eaten each item like a naturally thin person.

10. After you've tasted every item on the plate once, put your fork down, pause a moment, and look at the food again. Which of the foods were 10s for you, and what numbers would you give the other items?

11. Check your level of hunger before you continue. How much has your hunger level changed since you started?

12. Before you continue, do something your mother told you never to do—play with your food.

Rearrange it into a picture of something or make a design out of it.
Mash or mix it up.
Pick up a piece of food and while holding it a foot or two over your plate, "bomb" some target on your plate.

As you play with your food, listen to the voices in your head. If they try to get you to stop, thank them for their advice and keep going until you get tired of playing with your food.

Before you start eating again, pick up your plate and smell the foods again. What difference do you notice from the first time you smelled your food and now? Is the food starting to lose some of its emotional charge and become just food?

(Smelling the food on your plate is not recommended when you are in public.)

13. Continue the meal to satisfy your remaining hunger. Eat slowly, smell each bite before putting it into your mouth, and put your fork down before beginning to chew. Eat only the remaining foods on the plate that are 7s, 8s, 9s, or 10s for you.

14. As you complete the meal, keep checking your level of hunger. If you're not sure whether your body is at level 5, (not hungry) give yourself permission to eat three more bites, then stop for a moment, check your hunger level again, and continue if still hungry.

15. This next step may be very hard for you. Just keep breathing and stay in touch with what you are feeling and thinking.

When you reach "not hungry," pick up your plate, carry it to the garbage can, and very slowly discard the remaining food. Say good-bye to the food and thank it for giving itself to you. Notice how you feel about throwing food away instead of stuffing it into your body.

16. After each meal spend about five minutes just being with yourself and your experience. Write down your impressions of what eating like a naturally thin person was like for you after each meal. Write down what your body is experiencing and next what your mind is experiencing. Is the fat person talking to you? After each meal write down what your voice saying to you?

Meal #1:

Meal #2:

Meal #3:

17. After each meal is complete, refer to the list of things that you wanted to accomplish today. Pick the one which is the most important or the one that you most would like to do. Begin to work on that project.

18. After your first meal, instead of throwing any left over food away, wrap some of the parts worth saving for tomorrow.

19. Do the following exercise before going to sleep tonight.

EXERCISE

Write out how you feel about the work you did on your list of incompletions between meals today. Was it easy? fun? a chore? Did you feel like you won with any of them? Congratulate yourself below for what you accomplished.

20. As you fall asleep tonight, reflect on the experience of your naturally thin day. Congratulate yourself for letting your naturally thin person be in control as much as possible.

In Chapter 9 we'll talk about making the choice between the Diet Mentality and the Thin Mentality. Now that you've had an opportunity to experience what it might be like for you to be naturally thin, you'll be clearer about the choice you'll want to make. Before we reach the crossroads, I want to discuss in the next chapter why you might decide to choose fat over thin. As you'll see, the decision is not as clear-cut as it may at first appear.

Chapter 7

WHY YOU MIGHT STILL CHOOSE FAT OVER THIN

ARE YOU REALLY READY?

Wanting something and being committed to having it are two very different things. We want a lot of things, but we can only count on winding up with what we are committed to having.

When you are committed to something, you can measure your commitment by your daily actions and the results you are producing. If you are committed to your relationship, you do whatever it takes to make the relationship work. If you are committed to your children, they get taken care of, no matter how you are feeling. The question is, are you committed to becoming a naturally thin person and if not, how do you become committed?

The first question is harder to answer than you might first imagine. I know you probably "want" to be naturally thin, but the question is, are you committed? Are you ready to start producing daily results and taking daily actions toward becoming naturally thin?

Yes: No: Not yet: Not sure:

If you know that you are not fully committed yet or that you are not sure, how do you become committed? Think of those areas in your life where you are now committed. Maybe you can say absolutely that you are committed to your work, your relationship, or your children. How did you do that?

If you think about how you became committed for long, you will probably say something like, "I wanted to," or "I liked doing it." That's fine, except you probably "want to be" and "would like being" naturally thin.

I suggest that commitment shows up for most people like the flu. One moment they don't have it and the next they do. It is like they caught something. All fine and good, except you probably don't want to sit around waiting to catch the commitment to being naturally thin. You may be a patient person, but not that patient.

How can you become committed right now? Some say that if you say you are committed enough times with enough feeling, that you soon will be. For me, this idea worked on petty items, but when it came to being naturally thin, losing all of my weight, and keeping it off forever, this technique did not work.

I say that the commitment to being a naturally thin person comes from moving forward toward your goal until you are at the point of no return, until it is just as hard for you to turn back as it is to go forward. How do you get to the point of no return?... One step at a time.

First you say you are going to do something that will move you toward naturally thin and away from the diet mentality. Next, you do it. Then you say you are going to do something else, and you do that.

A friend of mine, Steve, told me a story about an old man he knew. One day Steve asked him how he had accomplished a particular goal that he had reached in his lifetime. The old man said, "It is easy. You 'hey', then you 'hook.' "

Steve asked what "you 'hey', you 'hook' " meant. With much effort, the old man stood up. He put one foot in front of the other and said, "You, 'hey.' " Then he moved the other foot forward and said, "Then, you 'hook.' " He began to pick up a little speed and each time he moved a step forward, he would say, "Hey! Hook! Hey! Hook!"

After you move forward far enough, you reach the point of no return and you are committed. The question now is, how do you move forward in this area of becoming naturally thin? What constitutes a step forward?

You make a promise that will move yourself forward as a naturally thin person and then you keep that promise. In other words, when you say that you are going to do something by a certain time, you do it.

This may sound easy, but look at your history of keeping your word in the area of your weight and your eating. How will you be able to keep promises in an area where you have always failed before? Why have you been able to keep promises in most other areas of your life, but never in this one?

This is a serious problem. Imagine that you had a job for a couple of years and that you got paid every Friday as soon as you walked in the door.

One Friday morning you walked in and your boss was standing there and said, "Good Morning! I know that you get paid every Friday morning, but this morning I am not going to pay you. I have this really great story about why you aren't going to get paid today, would you like to hear it?" What would you say? Probably that you would rather have your money than hear his story, right?

What if your boss continued to tell you this very sad story that was so good that he convinced you that even though you weren't getting paid as promised, you should go on to work anyway? On Monday morning when you walked in to work and saw your boss at the front door, what would be different about your relationship with him from this point on?

* Would you trust him as much as you had before he broke his promise to pay you?

* Would you respect him the same, more, or less than before?

* Do you imagine that you will be going out of your way in the future to do more or less than is demanded of you?

Your answers most likely are that you would trust and respect him less than before and that you would be less supportive of him and your work than you were before he broke his promise to you.

The reason for this is that when anyone breaks a promise about anything, he or she can count on losing trust, respect, and future support, no matter how good the reason for breaking the promise was. Each broken promise will lead to a greater loss of trust, respect, and support.

Given all of the promises that you have broken to yourself and others regarding losing weight and your eating, is it any wonder that you have lost a great deal of self respect? Is it hard to imagine supporting yourself one more time with no hesitation whatsoever in this area of your weight and eating?

KEEP   BREATHING

It is not as bad as you think. Let's look at the source of the problem. Why is it that you don't keep your promises in the area of your weight and eating even thought you do in other areas? Is it some form of selective brain damage, . . . do you not really want to lose weight, . . . or is there a more logical reason? I say that not keeping your word in the area of weight and eating is because of the diet mentality that you have been practicing.

If someone wanted to cleverly sabotage you, what kind of promises would you suppose he or she would ask you to make? They would not be impossible promises, because that would not be very clever, would it?

But, what would happen if you were asked to make promises that were just big promises? Not impossible promises, but only promises that if you were feeling very strong, clear, focused, and committed at every moment, you could accomplish. Something like:

    * Promise to go on and succeed on one of the 26,000 diets where 199 out of every 200 fail to lose their weight and keep it off.

    * Promise never to eat chocolate or one of your other favorite forbidden foods for the next five years.

    * Promise to lose 20 pounds in the next 30 days.

Are these big promises? What if you didn't eat chocolate for twelve whole weeks and then you had just one bite? What if you lost 10 pounds in the next thirty days? What did you do? You broke your promises. You would begin the vicious cycle of beating yourself up, trusting and respecting yourself less, and being even more unwilling to support yourself in doing anything else.

WHAT IS THE SOLUTION?

What is the solution? Don't say, "Don't make any promises." Without a promise, nothing happens. Most of our promises are not formal. We say something like, "I'll take care of that." Making smaller promises isn't the answer either. You need to start off with "baby" promises, promises that no matter what, you can be counted on to keep. As fragile as you are in this area of keeping your word about your weight and your eating, you need to make sure that you get a few wins under your belt. Baby steps forward are better than failures at this point.

What is a baby promise? All promises include a time frame. A specific and easily measurable time and date. The more vague your promises, the harder it will be to figure out if you kept them or not. Here are a few baby promises that you could make that would move you forward:

* Look ahead and promise to read two more pages within the next ten minutes.

* Promise to eat one meal tomorrow following rule number one...eating only if you are hungry.

* Promise to invite someone to be your partner in losing weight along with you by the time you go to bed tomorrow.

Write down your promise on a piece of paper and stick it in this book. Writing things down makes them more real. When you complete your promise, stop and really acknowledge yourself for doing what you said you would do. Don't worry if your diet mentality voice says something like, "Who cares! That's no big deal. Anyone could do that." Just thank your voice for sharing and continue to praise yourself until you feel acknowledged. At that point, thank yourself for the acknowledgment and revel in the warm feelings of accomplishment.

Why should you bother to take the time to acknowledge yourself for keeping your word and taking a small step forward? Because it completes that last promise and opens up the opportunity for your next promise.

CAUTION!

Do not get cocky and put on your promise shoes and go into a promising frenzy. Be very careful that your next promise is one that you will accomplish no matter what. Overcome any enthusiasm and excitement you may have picked up and make another baby promise. At some point you will get much stronger at keeping your word and will want to swing out with bigger promises. We will cover that subject in the last chapter.

AN "UP WITH WHICH
I WILL NOT PUT"

For years I have been interested in finding out why some smokers quit and stay off cigarettes and why others do not. The problem of smoking seems to be related in some way to overeating. I received many letters from people telling me that they had used *DIETS DON'T WORK* to not only lose their weight, but also to stop smoking.

Whenever I run across a smoker who has stopped smoking for over two years, I ask them whether they still feel like a smoker who is on some kind of smoking diet, or do they consider themselves a non–smoker? Do they still want to smoke or have they gotten to that point where they don't even like smoking anymore? Is it hard for them to breathe when they are around smoke and do they find the smell of smoke to be stale and offensive? Once a person reaches that status and identity of non–smoker, they almost never begin smoking again.

Getting to the point where you don't like the feeling of being bloated, the loss of energy, and the heaviness from overeating is one of the signs that you are well on your way to being naturally thin. How do you get to that point? How is becoming naturally thin similar to the way smokers become non–smokers?

Ask a person who has successfully stopped smoking and has become a non-smoker if they had ever tried to stop smoking before their last successful try and what made them make it the last time? When I have asked this question, the consistent theme of the answers that I got back was, "I wasn't willing to put up with smoking any longer!"

Are you still willing to put up with overeating as a response to feelings you are not willing to confront, or for any other reason? Do you still procrastinate in finding and using a more nurturing response to the triggers that get you to overeat? Are you going to be able to get to that place where overeating is an "up with which you will not put?"

I'm not trying to rush you. You need to trust the process you will choose to become naturally thin. Do what is best for you when you are ready, not when someone else is ready.

It took many people several years after they read *DIETS DON'T WORK* to be in a frame of mind to give up overeating and become naturally thin. The only right time to make that decision is when you are ready.

Do you think you are ready now? If not, have you a guess at the date you will be ready? Write out below what you are thinking right now. Just let all the thoughts you are having flow out. Get an extra notebook or diary and begin to use it to keep a diary of your thoughts, the conversations you have with yourself about your progress

toward being naturally thin. Using a diary or
journal every day is an effective way to begin to
spot, get out in the open, and turn around those
negative conversations that sometimes rage inside your head. Many times just saying something negative on paper is a good way to become
objective about it and let it go. So, what are you
thinking?

A non–smoker in Canada once gave me a great
thought to think about. When I asked her what
was different about the last time she quit smoking, she said, "I quit quiting."

That sounded fascinating, but after trying to
figure it out for a few moments, I asked her what
she meant? She said that she had quit smoking
many times before. This last time she made a
promise to herself. She would quit only this one
last time. If she so much as smoked even one
puff of one cigarette ever again, she would return
to smoking and never attempt to quit again. She
was sick and tired of promising to quit and
breaking her word to herself. She took a final
stand on this one last promise. Every time she

thought about smoking one more cigarette, she would decide whether that one cigarette was worth spending the rest of her life smoking or not. As far as I know, she is still a nonsmoker.

ARE YOU WILLING TO LEAVE YOUR CURRENT WEIGHT?

Are you sick and tired yet of overeating? Are you ready to let it go, or do you need a few more feeding frenzies?

Changing your weight permanently and becoming a naturally thin person can be a traumatic experience. Imagine shaving your head. Would you feel different? How easy would it be for you to begin to identify yourself and interact with people as a person with a shaved head? Would you feel comfortable?

Being naturally thin and losing your weight may be a bigger adjustment than you think. You will not only have to give up overeating as a response to all of your triggers, you will also have to think of yourself as a naturally thin person who does not use eating to deal with your feelings.

What are the advantages of weighing what you do now? What would you have to give up when you are naturally thin? Please write your thoughts below.

Have you thought about all of the clothes you will have to alter or get rid of because they will be too big? Are you ready to spend the money fixing or buying new clothes?

Losing weight and feeling better about yourself usually means looking more attractive. Who will you attract? I don't want to sound pessimistic, but if you are a woman, more than likely it will not be Tom Cruise. What if it is some creep that has been living under a rock who wants to paw and drool on you? Or worse, someone who is also attractive to you. What if you are in a committed relationship? Won't that cause problems? Will you be able to say, "Thank you. That's the nicest compliment I've had all day" and walk away?

What about losing your weight and still being rejected? Being overweight may have given you a justification for any rejection you may have suffered. You didn't like yourself very much either, but if that reason is gone, can you deal with continued rejection?

If you enjoyed the attention you got while losing weight, what is going to happen when people begin to take your weight loss for granted? What will you do to get the attention that you require? Gain the weight back?

WILL IT BE WORTH IT?

Will what it is going to take for you to become a naturally thin person and stay that way for the rest of your life be worth your time and effort?

There is nothing wrong with being overweight. Much of the disease attributed to excess weight has more to do with excessive overeating and stress than from the weight itself. If you can't walk up a flight of stairs without getting out of breath, don't confuse being overweight with being out of condition. Most naturally thin people who aren't physically fit cannot climb stairs without being winded either.

The question to ask yourself is this. How will being naturally thin change your life? What specific measurable difference is being naturally thin going to make in your life? Write your answer below.

Are your reasons good enough to get you to do whatever it is going to take to become and stay naturally thin? What if it takes as long to reverse your weight problem as it took you to create it? Will you practice being naturally thin for as long and as patiently as you have practiced overeating?

Will you allow yourself to be surrounded by supportive people who also want to live the rest of their lives as naturally thin?

If necessary, are you going to be willing to work with a therapist or Diets Don't Work Trained Consultant in order to find the source of what is triggering you to overeat or to discover other solutions to your trigger eating?

Chapter 8

MAKING THE CHOICE NOW

TRUST THE PROCESS

I have talked to a lot of people about the results they achieved after reading *DIETS DON'T WORK*. Some, like my wife Leah, lost weight immediately and had an easy time keeping it off.

Others took a very winding path. Some spent several years going back and forth until one day everything clicked and the weight and overeating dropped away.

By this time you should have a feeling about what the future holds for you. You may be afraid, but I would bet that you know right now if being naturally thin is in your future.

The question is, will you stick with it...no matter how long it takes or how much support you need?

HITTING BOTTOM

At Alcoholics Anonymous they usually find it is a waste of time to talk to alcoholics until they have hit bottom. Only then is the person willing to listen and take action.

RAISING THE BOTTOM

If overeating and weight are to be ended as a problem for everyone by the year 2000 A.D., you and I are going to have to find some way to raise the bottom. One of the strategies to raise the bottom is to raise people's consciousness, to let everyone know that there is a possibility to have their eating and their bodies exactly the way they want. The missing ingredient for most people is knowledge.

Your present behavior is based on your past knowledge and experiences. Our behavior shapes us. Unless we change the knowledge that determines our behavior, we will continue to act the same way as in the past and wind up with the same results.

Naturally thin behavior means learning information which we do not now possess. The information we require, however, is not that hard to come by.

What do ex-overeaters do when confronted by situations which urge them to overeat? The answer is to do the same thing that a naturally thin person would do if confronted by the same situation.

Don't overeaters and naturally thin people think differently? Yes! But, the good news is that if you were taught how to overeat, you can also be taught to think and thereby react in a naturally thin way.

An example of thinking like a naturally thin person could be a situation of being under stress. What if you were a naturally thin person and you were involved in a stressful situation of some kind? Let's say that you did everything that you knew how to do to remedy the situation and then, when the day was over, you went home.

When the naturally thin person got home, what would they do? Would they head for the refrigerator and start overeating? No?

Why not? Because overeating does not occur to them as a solution to their stress. They do not rely on this behavior as a solution, no more than an overeater would go home and drink two gallons of water in a pressure situation.

How do you go about eliminating the "reality" of overeating as a solution to your problems? Begin to THINK! Before you begin to eat, stop. Take a breath. Describe what has happened, what you are feeling, and what you are about to do to remedy this situation.

(Example: "At work today, nothing I did made the problem that I was faced with go away. I feel very tense. I am a level 5 in my hunger level. I want to eat until my tension and worry are gone.")

Next, describe what will happen if you eat.

(Example: "I will start calming down as I eat more and more. Then I will start to feel bloated and heavy. I will begin to feel tired and sluggish. Then I will feel fat and start to beat myself up because I said that I want to eat like a naturally thin person but I failed.")

Next, describe what would happen if you do not eat as a response to your stressful situation. (Example: "My mind will keep going over and over my worry. I will feel incompetent and powerless. I might feel better if I exercised, but I will probably be too tired to make myself do that. I could go to a movie or lay down and take a nap. Maybe I can call a friend to go for a walk with me so that I could talk about what was bothering me as we walked? I could walk until I had resolved the problem or until I felt exhausted enough to come home and sleep. A shower or bath might wash away some of the stress I am feeling. I could even write a letter to myself or write in my daily journal and vent all the thoughts that keep running through my mind. Maybe by writing down my problems and their possible solutions, I might get things in perspective again.")

What I have described are two very different scenarios. On your path to being a naturally thin person, you may be successful sometimes reacting as a naturally thin person and at other times not. The important thing is to forgive yourself when you fail. Keep asking yourself, "Can you love yourself for doing that?"

Another thing to do is to acknowledge to yourself over and over—until you have gone past the point of comfort—everything that you do right. Even if you only succeed for a few minutes, acknowledge your progress. Magnify it. Dwell on it. Remember it. Write it down. Go to bed thinking about your progress and imagine repeating and expanding on it in the future. WHAT YOU FOCUS ON WILL EXPAND. Focus on what you want more of, not on what you don't want.

WHAT'S YOUR HURRY?

Would now be a good time for you to stop for a while? If you are not ready to take the plunge into the naturally thin life by now, it may be a sign for you to stop reading now and start over at the beginning of this book or switch over to *DIETS DON'T WORK*.

Do what feels right. At this point, listen to your heart, not your head. Your heart tugs on you gently and whispers in your ear, urging you to go in the direction that is right for you. Your head, or mind, usually screams impatiently at you.

When confronted by a fork in the road, especially when a lot is at stake, most of us feel the sensation of fear in our stomach, chest, throat, or knees. Sometimes our tendency is to freeze, to do nothing, or to run away.

On your way to becoming a naturally thin person, the best way to handle fear is to imagine your fear as if it were a beach ball. If you let it stop you, it will grow. The ball of fear will become so large that trying to move it will paralyze you.

The better way to deal with fear is to carefully tuck the ball of fear under your arm, take a deep breath, and take action. As long as you keep breathing and hang on to your ball of fear tightly, you will start to notice that your fear will begin to get smaller and smaller.

Can you recall a time when you let your fear stop you from taking action? Briefly describe the situation.:

Do you remember how you felt afterwards? Did the fear rob you of all your power and grow to such a size that you felt dwarfed by it?

Can you recall a time when you took a risk even though you felt afraid? Briefly describe the situation:

Did your risk pay off? How?

Can you recall what happened to your fear?
Did it disappear? How big did you feel afterwards?

TAKING A RISK IS THE FASTEST WAY TO
RECONNECT YOU TO YOUR POWERFUL SIDE.
Now may be the right time for you to turn back
and slowly start over, or are you ready to plunge
ahead into the unknown? Trust yourself. Listen

to your heart. Turning back or forging ahead will both be a risk. Do whatever you need to do. Forging ahead may seem scary, but if the faint whisper of your heart says go for it, plunge ahead and make your decision work.

Even a wrong choice is far better than no choice at all. Making no choice is like staring at the blinking hold button on a telephone. No matter how long you stare at that button, nothing happens until somebody does something. If you make the wrong choice, if you pick up the wrong line, at least you know the direction not to go in. You can then re-choose.

One of the exercises in the Diets Don't Work Weekend Workshop is to listen to your inner voice and to take risks. IF IT SCARES YOU, DO IT! For two days the participants learn to keep stepping outside their normal boundaries. They learn how to be naturally thin in an environment as challenging as they will probably ever have to face in real life. If they can react as a naturally thin person in the workshop, they can do the same in the real world.

Start right now to begin practicing living outside your normal boundaries. Instead of waiting until you lose your weight, start to take risks now. Challenge the naturally thin person inside of you. Grasp your fear tightly and go after your dreams. What have you got to lose?

EXERCISE:

"These are the things that I am afraid to do or say until I am naturally thin:"

"These are the specific actions I will begin to take and the exact time I will start:"

PART 3

LIVING THE
NATURALLY THIN LIFE

Chapter 9

HOW TO HAVE A
BREAKTHROUGH, RIGHT NOW

First of all, don't make the same mistake that most people, including "professionals" in the weight loss business, make. Be sure you are able to make the important distinctions between:

(1) Eating too much,
(2) Exercise, and
(3) Nutrition.

1. Eating too much: *DIETS DON'T WORK* and *DIETS STILL DON'T WORK* are about eliminating habitual overeating from your life. If you stop eating too much, you will shed excess weight.

2. Exercise: The purpose of exercise is to be physically fit, to feel and look your best. You can be physically fit and still be overweight.

It takes thirty minutes of aerobic dancing to burn off twelve corn chips. Does it take anyone you know thirty minutes to eat twelve corn chips? Probably not. The bottom line is that the fastest exerciser cannot burn up the number of calories that even the slowest overeater can take in.

Most everyone would like to be physically fit and feel and look better, but what kind of exercise is the most fun and will be the most valuable for you? When should you consider starting an exercise program?

I have seen thousands of people lose weight using the principles of *DIETS DON'T WORK*. I noticed that once people began to eat like a naturally thin person, they began to feel better and have more energy. It feels good to stop overeating and even better to begin to lose weight without deprivation or struggle. "What can I do to even feel better than this?" they would begin to ask.

Exercise! Exercise not only uses up some of that new found energy that you will be feeling, exercise will also inspire you to be more conscious of eating like a naturally thin person.

Some of the exercise benefits you will discover are:

A. Exercise is an effective way to rid yourself of stress and can prevent overeating caused by stress.

B. Exercise releases pent up energy and frustrations.

C. Exercise causes almost immediate improvement in the way you look. Exercise tightens and tones loose flabby muscles. Losing inches becomes the motivation to exercise even more.

D. Exercising allows you to use time, once spent overeating, in a productive and fun way.

E. Exercising is a great way to meet and receive the support of other people who are also motivated to be physically fit, feel their best, and lead healthy lives.

3. Nutrition: What's the purpose of nutrition? To be thin or to be healthy? Both would be nice, but the bottom line of nutrition is to be healthy. Being overweight does not automatically mean that you are unhealthy.

Everyone would like to be as healthy as possible and feel better, but what kind of nutrition program would be the most fun and valuable for you? When should you consider starting to work on your nutrition?

Watching thousands of people lose weight using *DIETS DON'T WORK*, I noticed that once people began to eat in a naturally thin way and began to become physically fit, they began to feel much better and have more energy. It feels great to stop overeating, to begin to lose weight, and to start becoming physically fit.

"What can we do to even feel better than this?" they would ask.

Nutrition! Eat more nutritious foods. But, WHEN to start is a critical factor. If people got in a hurry and started too soon or if the nutrition program took too much effort and was too hard, the "diet mentality" was quickly triggered. They began to feel deprived and shortly thereafter they would begin to binge on junk food once again. What was the answer?

The answer was to wait until Rule #2 of eating like a naturally thin person began to become a problem. The problem was when people got to a point in eating like a naturally thin person where they began to have a hard time figuring out EXACTLY WHAT WOULD SATISFY THEM.

They would know for sure that they were definitely hungry, but they could not think of anything that they were especially drawn to eat which would satisfy them more than anything else. Was the problem that they were not really hungry?

For a while, I thought so, but then I saw what was happening. **THE FREEDOM TO EAT EXACTLY WHAT TOTALLY SATISFIES HUNGER WILL TAKE THE IMPORTANCE AWAY FROM ALL FORBIDDEN FOODS.** One food becomes just as unimportant as another. What you eat begins not to matter and if what you eat is not important, why not kill two birds with one stone? WHY NOT EAT SOMETHING THAT IS HIGH IN NUTRITIONAL VALUE AT THE SAME TIME YOU SATISFY YOUR BODY'S HUNGER?

This method of approaching nutrition has a great deal of freedom in it and explained why so many of the people that I had followed up on had begun to eat at higher and higher levels of nutrition. The amazing thing was that most people achieved healthy eating almost without any conscious effort.

Donna, of Northern California, said:

"I am now wearing tight pants which a few years ago were only a dream. Before reading *DIETS DON'T WORK*, I had gotten up to a high of 320 pounds.

"When I first got married, even though I weighed only 130 pounds at 5'3", everybody said that I was fat. I began to think of myself as fat even though I wasn't. I did every weight loss program that there was and either quit before losing my weight or gained my weight back shortly after losing it.

"I weighed 289 pounds when I first picked up *DIETS DON'T WORK*. I knew God had sent me the answer. I lost 90 pounds over the first 18 months. I wasn't dieting or feeling deprived. It was wonderful. Then, everything came to a slow halt. I was standing still. I didn't know if it was because my body needed more time or if I was beginning to slightly overeat again.

"I began to see a therapist who was recommended to me and, even though I began to find out a lot of things about myself, my weight stayed the same.

"Once in a while I would talk to one of the Diets Don't Work staff over the phone and have a private consulting session. I discovered that the DIETS DON'T WORK program had not only given me the kind of freedom with food that I had never experienced before, it had given me more freedom than was comfortable for me to handle. I needed less freedom, but I needed enough structure to keep me awake to the principles of *DIETS DON'T WORK*. With the support of my consultant at Diets Don't Work and my therapist, I returned to Weight Watchers.

"At first the Weight Watchers environment was strange. I had to listen at two levels to what was going on. On one level I could hear how many of the people there were still operating out of the 'Diet Mentality.' On the other hand, I had a feeling of tremendous support. The eating program at Weight Watchers was, of course, full of well balanced meals and healthy types of foods. Most of the time I was relieved not to have to decide exactly what I wanted, but to just eat what was on the menu for that meal. By following the *DIETS DON'T WORK* principles I had learned, I was able to 'eat EXACTLY what satisfied me' at every meal.

"Sometimes I would have a craving for a particular food such as a hot fudge sundae at Baskin-Robbins. This was certainly not on my Weight Watchers program, but I followed each of the four rules for eating outlined in the *DIETS DON'T WORK* technique. By the next meal, I was right back to eating my WEIGHT WATCHERS program and still following the principles of *DIETS DON'T WORK*. All during this time, I NEVER FELT DEPRIVED!

"I have lost a total of 40 more pounds over the last year and am a 'Naturally Thin Person' thanks to *DIETS DON'T WORK*.

"I had done Weight Watchers and therapy before, but the missing ingredient for me was the *DIETS DON'T WORK* philosophy."

Donna's story underlines an important fact. Overeating and nutrition are two different conversations. They should be talked about and tackled separately.

Which first? If immediate health factors are not a pressing issue for you, the goal of losing weight and stopping overeating will probably be your top priority. If your doctor has no objections, I recommend that you address and master eating like a naturally thin person first.

I am not saying that nutrition is not important. People are most effective, however, when they first deal with the issue which is most important.

Remember, the purpose of nutrition is to be as healthy as you can possibly be. Being healthy is an important goal, but if you are suffering because of your weight or overeating, you most likely will realize that until the weight and overeating is handled, you will not be very motivated to work on improving your nutrition.

A BREAKTHROUGH IN "WITHHOLD EATING"

In Chapter Four, I talked about "Withholds" as one of the major reasons for people overeating. Most readers assume that I am talking about everyone but them.

Many of the people in the Diets Don't Work Weekend Workshop also doubted that they had any withholds that were causing them to overeat. Almost every one of them reported that they lost weight from using the following withhold process. Try it at least five times before you decide for yourself.

Withholds cause a great deal of tension and stress in the withholder. Withholds can also cause stress and tension if you are the person being withheld from. Can you recall the tension you feel if you sense that something is being held back from you?

In order to get some relief from the uncomfortable body sensations that this tension and stress causes, the withholder, or the person being withheld from, usually finds himself or herself either overeating or in some cases overdrinking.

THE SOLUTION IS TO ELIMINATE THE WITHHOLD. I created a method that makes eliminating withholds easier than you can imagine. Most of the time you do not even have to talk directly to the person with which you have the withhold.

According to thousands of people who attended the Diets Don't Work Weekend Workshops, the following technique was one of the most valuable things that they learned in the workshop. The technique worked not only for losing weight and keeping it off, but also for making a big difference in their relationships and lives.

You will probably not want to try this technique. Neither did they. They would ask every question possible in order to try to stall for time. They would become confused and not be able to understand the instructions. Some would get sleepy. Anything to get out of trying this technique.

I am telling you this because as a reader of *DIETS STILL DON'T WORK*, you will have an easy time avoiding this technique. All you have to do is close the book and walk away or just skip to the next chapter. Please don't!

I am promising you thousands of dollars worth of value if you learn to use this very simple technique. To skip over it will be ripping yourself off and undermining your chances of becoming naturally thin.

Just try it five times. If you follow the instructions you could lose as much as five pounds in the process.

WITHHOLD PROCESS

Put a check mark by each of the following steps as you complete each one. Take them one at a time.

___A. Go back to Chapter 4 and look under the heading called "THE BIG TWELVE." Item number 4 had an exercise which asked you to list thoughts, feelings, or information that you had withheld from different groups of people. Go back to that section now and find that list of withholds. If for some reason you did not complete your lists, please do so before continuing.

__B. Next, read over your list of withholds in Chapter 4 and put a small check mark by the one which would be the easiest and the one that would be the hardest for you to disclose to the person with which you had the withhold.

__C. Choose which one you would be willing to communicate. The bigger the withhold, the bigger the result you will produce with this exercise. Take as big of a risk as you feel you can take.

__D. Find someone who is willing to pretend to be the person that you have the withhold from. You may do this exercise over the phone, but, it will be more effective if you do it in person

__E. Give your substitute these instructions:

__1. First tell him who he is pretending to be. If he does not know the person, fill him in quickly on background information: age, relationship to you, basic personality, how the person interacts with you normally, and how the person might interact with you in a somewhat stressful situation. Don't tell him anything about the withhold that you are about to bring up.

__2. Have him notice what thoughts or feelings he is having while pretending to be the person he is playing.

__3. Tell him to say whatever occurs to him or express whatever feelings that arise in him while doing his part. During the first five steps of this process he can for the most part just go along with you. When you get to step six, his job is to be as aggressive as he can pretend to be. Tell him to hold nothing back. He should verbally attack you and try to say every mean and hurtful thing that he can make up. During step six, he does most of the talking. He should hit you with only one thing at a time. After you respond to what he says, he can say the next thing that occurs to him

__4. Let him know that you may "direct" him from time to time if you think the response he is giving you is not one you would get from the actual person.

__5. The main thing that you are asking him to do is to play along. Tell him to be as spontaneous as possible. Remind him to say whatever thoughts occur to him and be influenced by whatever feelings he gets during the exercise. Under no circumstance should he take pity on you or be reasonable with you. Even if he has to make something up, his job is to try to make you feel as bad as possible.

___F. Follow one by one these next six steps. Pretend that your substitute is really the actual person that you have the withhold from. Try to feel all of the feelings you would have if he were really the person.

START THE EXERCISE:

1. TIME: Tell your substitute that you have something to talk to him about and ask him if he has five minutes (an exact amount of time) to talk to you right now?

If he says yes, continue. If he hesitates or says no, tell him that you have something very important to tell him and ask him for a time when he will have five minutes. Make an appointment.

2. "THIS IS HARD!": Let him know with as few words as possible, but with as much feeling and expression as you can muster that, "This is very difficult for you," or "What you are about to tell him is hard for you to say."

3. FEARS: Next let him know all the fears you have about telling him what you are about to tell him. Don't give any hints or direct information

about what it is that you are going to say to him. You could say, "I'm afraid to tell you this because:

* you will probably be mad at me.
* you may never trust me again.
* you're probably going to think that I'm being unreasonable.
* you'll think I'm blowing things out of proportion, or that I'm being silly.
* it will hurt your feelings.
* you'll think that I shouldn't feel the way I do.
* you won't love me anymore, you may want to leave me, fire me, or hit me.
* you'll think I'm stupid, irresponsible, careless."

Tell him all of your fears without revealing any clues about what you are going to talk about. If he tries to rush you to tell him what you are talking about, just keep saying, "I'm getting to that."

4. IDEAL RESPONSE: After you have completed revealing all of your fears, ask if he would promise to do or not do the following things. (At this point you may ASK for anything that you want, no matter how unreasonable. It does not matter if he agrees or not, the important thing is that you ASK and get either a yes, no, or maybe from him.)

Ask for everything that you want as clearly and straightforward as possible. Some things you might want to ask for before you tell him the withhold are:

* not to interrupt you while you are talking. It may make you lose your train of thought and you will forget to tell him something. When you are finished, he can ask you anything or say anything that he wants to.

* to do nothing else while you tell him what you are about to tell him. You would like his full attention.

Some of the things you might ask for that will apply to after you have told him your withhold are:

* a request for him to promise not to be mad at you, scream at you, hit you, or leave you.

* request that he promise to try to forgive you, understand how you feel, put himself in your shoes.

* tell him not to believe anything you are about to say. All you want to do is to get a lot of negative energy off of your chest and you do not want to be inhibited in any way. You may want

to scream, yell, pound your fists, jump up and down, exaggerate, or be irresponsible. You are asking him to just listen to you and try to understand how you feel. You might suggest that he pretend he is watching a television show. In other words, he should not take anything you say personally or even think you are talking about him. (This instruction is very useful if you are really angry at someone. It allows the person to "hear" what you are saying without shutting down or getting defensive. If you say everything that you think and feel while expressing yourself fully, all of the energy can be released from your withhold and you will feel complete, no matter what the person's response is.)

Most of the time it will not matter if your substitute agrees or declines your request. The important thing is that you ask.

You may, of course, have a nonnegotiable request. If you demand certain conditions and he refuses to give you total reassurance that your conditions be met, you do not have to continue. For example, you might ask him to take the phone off the hook for five minutes. If he refuses because he is expecting a very important call, ask for another time when he will not be busy.

5. "WHAT I DON'T WANT TO TELL YOU IS:"

This is the step where you tell him exactly what you have been withholding from him.

Take a deep breath and START AT THE BEGINNING OF THE STORY. Too many times, you forget that although the story you are about to tell is very familiar to you, your real life listener may have forgotten all about it. Briefly go back to some neutral period prior to the incident and, covering the high points, bring him up to the moment of the incident. For example, one of the participants in the weekend workshop told about delivering a withhold to her husband. She started with:

"Do you remember the first time we met? You asked me for a date that night and by the end of the week you asked me to marry you. Do you remember that?

"We've been married two years now, does it seem that long to you?

"Do you recall, last week, when I asked you if it was all right with you if I bought some new clothes? We are going to that party tonight and I asked you if I could get something new to wear? You said O.K., as long as I didn't spend over $100, remember?

"Well, I went shopping and got exactly what I wanted, but I spent more than $100. How much more? Oh, about triple; $297.50 to be exact. Are you mad at me for breaking my promise to you?"

6. LET HIM BE RIGHT: You may have thought that step number 5 was the hardest part of this process, but you were wrong. Many times we

are smart enough to prepare the person we are talking to before we drop a "withhold" bomb on him. The mistake we make is that we don't realize that even though we have said everything that we need to say, the conversation still is not complete. THE PERSON WE ARE TALKING TO HAS NOT SAID EVERYTHING THAT HE NEEDS TO SAY.

In order to make this a complete and successful communication, you have to make sure that the other person says EVERYTHING that he needs to say. In order to do this you must do three things.

First, keep asking him questions, such as, "How do you feel about that?" And, keep repeating, "Is there anything else?" until he has nothing else to say.

The second thing you need to do is to listen to every word, every tone in his voice, and watch every expression carefully.

Third, and the hardest thing that you must do is to agree with everything that he says as enthusiastically as possible. I don't mean lie to him, but if even one thing in a sentence is true, tell him that he is right about that part and let the rest slide. For example, if her husband had said, "You promised to spend only $100 and you knew all along you were going to spend more than that." If you didn't intend to spend over

$100, but did promise to spend only $100, you would agree with the part that was true and drop the rest. She would say, "You're right. I did promise to spend only $100." and then ask "Anything else?"

Don't argue. Don't defend yourself or try to justify what you did. If your partner says something that hurts you, tell the truth. Say, "Ouch! That really hurts when you say that . . . Anything else?"

If they accuse you of something that you did not do, don't argue that you didn't do it. Say, "I'm surprised that you think I would do that (or I'm surprised that you feel that way). Anything else?" Many times the best thing to say when you feel your partner is way off base is, "Mmmmm! I see. Anything else?"

Your job during this completion phase is to get him to pull every arrow out of his quiver and shoot it as deeply and painfully as he can into the most sensitive part of you. As he releases each arrow, keep breathing and open up wider each time for the next arrow. Don't defend. Don't argue. Don't try to be right or sarcastic. Take in all of the anger, distrust, resentment, hurt, until he is empty. Show as much sadness, hurt, or regret as possible. Do not show any righteousness, anger, or impatience. Once your substitute says everything that he or she can think of or make up, the process is complete.

After the process is complete using your substitute, check out how you feel. You will either feel a lot lighter or a lot heavier.

If you feel lighter, you are complete with the process. Check and see how many pounds lighter you feel? Write that number down here.

If you feel heavier, you have left something out while you were telling the withhold, or you resisted letting your substitute win when he was attacking you. Some piece of the truth was left out. Go back and do the process again. This time pretend to be the villain in your story instead of a victim or hero. (Tell the withhold as if you set the whole thing up on purpose. Find areas where you did something that may have caused or led up to the incident.)

You may feel like doing the process "live" with the actual person after your practice session with your substitute. If doing the process live would be too much of a risk or impossible to do, use your substitute to run through the process a few more times. You will know that the withhold is gone when you are not able to remember it any longer. Another sign that the withhold is gone is when there is no more energy left on the withhold when you think about delivering it live.

With small withholds, you do not always need a substitute to practice with before you deliver it live. But, if you have a juicy withhold, an emotional bomb, always use a substitute. Rehearse enough times to be ready for whatever happens.

Be careful when using this withhold process. Telling the truth WILL set you free, but it also can get you fired, hit, shot, divorced, and nailed to a cross.

On the side of letting go of every withhold that you have, think about this...Why would you want to be in a relationship with anyone to whom you can't tell the truth? Some of your withholds are probably keeping a bunch of unwanted pounds on your body. Can you afford to keep carrying them around?

Go back and practice the withhold process at least four more times on different items from your list in Chapter 4. As you think of more withholds, add them to your list. Write down the six steps on a piece of paper and refer to your notes as much as is needed.

Check off each withhold from your list as it disappears and write down the number of pounds lighter that you feel after getting rid of it.

Chapter 10

THE PHYSICAL TRANSITION

Beginning to act like a naturally thin person is a little like being set down on a strange planet. You don't know exactly how to act. It's an exciting new world, but what do you do next?

First of all, give yourself a lot of time to make the transition to naturally thin. You're on the verge of beginning a whole new life, and you need to be gentle and patient with yourself. Don't expect to wake up the first morning knowing everything you need to know to be a naturally thin person. This part of the naturally thin process is a time of transition, a time when you're moving from being a fat person to being a naturally thin person. Sometimes it takes a while.

As I was making the physical transition, I discovered several principles or techniques that supported the thin person and made it easier for the naturally thin part of me to emerge.

LEVELS OF HUNGER

Naturally thin people eat **only** when they're hungry and stop when they reach the feeling of being not hungry. As we discussed in "Thin For a Day," you'll need to be clear about when you're hungry and when you're not.

The following is an expanded explanation of the hunger scale:

1. You're wobbly and dizzy. You can hardly think. The fuel gauge of your body is empty. There's absolutely nothing in your tank. Most people have to go all day without food to get close to a level 1.

2. You're very hungry, but you could probably stagger to the dinner table. You're probably feeling irritable and cranky.

3. You are nice and hungry. The urge to eat is strong.

4. You're only a little hungry. Your body is sending messages that you might want to eat a little something.

4.9 Your hunger has almost totally disappeared. You may be just one bite away from not hungry.

5. "Not Hungry." You aren't hungry anymore. Your body has had what it needed and is satisfied. This is where naturally thin people stop eating.

5.1 You've put just a tiny bit more food into your body than it needs. You have crossed the line into overeating.

6. You're past being satisfied. You feel FULL. You are aware of a slightly bloated feeling in your body.

7. You're becoming uncomfortable. You're starting to feel as if your stomach has stretched a few inches. The bloat is starting to make you feel heavy.

8. You're more than full, and your stomach is starting to hurt. You almost wish you hadn't had that second helping.

9. Your body is screaming, "Get me out of here!" and the pain is setting in. It's absolutely no fun anymore. You feel as if they're going to have to put you on a truck and haul you away.

10. This is Thanksgiving Day full, when you have to roll yourself to the couch after dinner and all you can do is lay there. You didn't realize you were eating that much, and now you wish someone could cut it out of you. You hurt for hours and swear you won't eat again for a week.

If your hunger level is under five, you're feeding your naturally thin body. If it's over five, you're feeding your head. Only it's your body, not your head, that gets fat.

When people first start to work with the levels of hunger, they sometimes get a little confused. If you haven't experienced hunger in a long time and you feel the slightest body sensation, you may think you're at a 1. Actually you're probably closer to a 3 or a 4. Figuring out your level of hunger takes a little time and practice.

10
9
8
7
6
5—

4

3

2

1

Close your eyes and place your hands on your stomach. Ask your body if it's hungry. Is it a 4? a 3 1/2? a 5? Listen to what your body says. It can give you a lot of information if you learn its language. You may not have listened to it in quite a while except to berate it, so it may be shy. Listen again. The more you listen to your body, the more it will have to say.

EXERCISES (1 minute)

1. What is your level of hunger right now?

2. What would you guess your level of hunger usually is when you eat:?

Breakfast?:

Lunch?:

Dinner?:

3. What is usually your level of hunger when you stop eating?

Breakfast?:

Lunch?:

Dinner?:

"You Can Never Get Enough of What You Don't Really Want"*

(*Quote by Eric Hoffer)

The second principle of *DIETS DON'T WORK* is to eat exactly what you want, exactly what will satisfy you. For a naturally thin person, if it's not EXACTLY what he likes and wants, why should he eat it.

If you've been on lots of diets, you've probably been programed to ignore what you like and trained to eat dozens of foods you don't like. The whole idea of choosing food that is absolutely delicious and satisfying may be scary or unimaginable to you. Discovering exactly what

141

you like, what will satisfy you, what your 9s and 10s are, will be an exciting adventure. You will learn to look inside rather than outside yourself for clues on what to eat.

As you begin to choose foods that are 9s and 10s, you'll discover a funny thing. Many foods will remain a 10 for only a short period of time; their big attraction was probably that they were forbidden. Once you get enough of them, you'll find yourself wanting them only occasionally. Another thing you can expect is that your body is going to want to eat funny things at funny times. For instance, I got up one morning and asked my body what it wanted for breakfast. The dialogue went something like this:

Me: What do you want for breakfast this morning?

Body: Rocky Road ice cream from Baskin-Robbins.

Me: Come on. Are you crazy? Stop kidding around. What do you really want for breakfast?

Body: Rocky Road ice cream.

Me: Look, you don't understand. We're talking breakfast—eggs, toast, orange juice, cereal, stuff like that. What do you want?

Body: Rocky Road ice cream!

Me: You're crazy, I'm not listening to you anymore.

So I ate eggs, toast, orange juice, and cereal for breakfast. The only problem was that I wasn't satisfied afterward. My body still wanted Rocky Road ice cream. The next morning when I asked my body what it wanted, this is the dialogue that ensued:

Me: What do you want for breakfast this morning?
Body: Rocky Road ice cream.

Me: OK, but Baskin-Robbins doesn't open until 11:00 A.M.; you're going to have to wait until then.

Body: Fine. I'll wait.

At 11:00 A.M. I was waiting outside Baskin-Robbins with my nose pressed up against the glass. I bought my scoop of Rocky Road ice cream, ate it, and was totally satisfied. I didn't get hungry or eat again until 6:00 p.m.. That's all my body wanted. The first time, I had listened to the voice of my Diet Mentality: "Nobody eats ice cream for breakfast." The second time, I listened to my body, to my naturally thin self, and I ate exactly what I wanted and was satisfied. Do you begin to see the difference? You could just as easily find yourself wanting to eat breakfast foods for lunch or dinner. For example: "What do you want for dinner? A bowl of cereal with strawberries? Great!" IT TAKES A LOT LESS TO SATISFY YOU WHEN YOU'RE EATING EXACTLY WHAT YOU WANT. And if you watch naturally thin people, you'll see this principle at work.

NUTRITION

The biggest concern of most people when they think about following the rule "eat exactly what you want" has to do with nutrition. "What if I eat hot fudge sundaes and candy all of the time? That's what I usually want." You may think that you will go crazy with this much freedom, but IF you wait until you are hungry, if you are eating EXACTLY what you want and are ENJOYING every bite CONSCIOUSLY, your fears will prove to be unfounded.

"ICE CREAM DIET"

The popular "Ice Cream Diet" proved to me that we can lose interest in even our most

144

favorite food if we followed the *DIETS DON'T WORK* eating principles.

People in my health clubs began to tell me that they had found this great diet for people who loved ice cream. You just eat as much ice cream, any flavor, as you want at every meal. Nothing else. The first day they started out in heaven, but by the end of the day they were starting to slow down. The next day they waited until they were really hungry to eat. By the third day they were dreaming of plain lettuce and sick of the idea of eating another bite of ice cream.

"CRACKER JACK PERIOD"

Another example of how "eating exactly what you want" works comes from a story I read about an experiment carried on in an orphanage. The children in the orphanage were told that for thirty days they would not be restricted to the meals normally served. The dining room had been set up buffet style and they could go in anytime they were hungry and eat as much of anything as they wanted. A two way mirror was set up in the dining room so that the group of doctors conducting the experiment could monitor what and how much each child ate without the children knowing. One little boy drove them crazy. The first morning he walked into the dining room, got a plate, and looked over everything that was available. Then, he filled his plate with Cracker Jacks (caramel coated popcorn) and proceeded to eat until he could eat no more. At lunch, he got his plate and went directly to the Cracker Jacks without even looking at anything else. At dinner, he continued to do the same thing.

The doctors thought that this was the funniest thing that they had ever seen, but as each day passed, they began to stop laughing and started to worry. The little boy continued to eat nothing but Cracker Jacks at each meal. The doctors worried that the boy might get sick from eating only cracker jacks and they would get in trouble for what was now beginning to look like a bad idea.

Seven days went by and finally the boy stopped eating Cracker Jacks and began to eat other things. He began to drink milk, eat fruit, vegetables, and meat. At the end of the thirty days the doctors added up everything that the boy had eaten and averaged it out. To their surprise it averaged out to be a balanced diet.

You may go through your "Cracker Jack" period. Don't worry. As long as you wait until you are hungry, eat EXACTLY what you want, and consciously ENJOY every bite, this phase will quickly pass. You will begin to notice that you are starting to be drawn to eat things that make you feel your best as well as satisty your hunger.

As I covered in Chapter 9, once you get to the point where you are hungry and nothing particularly seems more important to eat than anything else, why not begin to eat the most nutritious foods possible? This point in your progress toward being naturally thin is the perfect time to begin to cut down on the amounts of oil, grease, butter, and salt that you eat and take in more fresh fruits and vegetables. The best thing that you could do at this point might be to attend classes in nutrition or work with a registered nutritionist who is familiar with the *DIETS DON'T WORK* principles.

You will have already started feeling better because you will be losing weight and will no longer be overeating. At this point, why not increase your level of nutrition to make yourself feel even better?

Being committed to a high level of nutrition in order to be as healthy as possible is an admirable goal. The mistake that most people make is that they try to introduce nutrition into their lives at a time when they are already feeling deprived. Any additional deprivation from trying to follow a strict nutritional program usually causes them to blow the whole program and revert to their old habits of overeating.

THE RULE OF THREE

What if you're halfway through a meal, and you can't tell whether or not you're hungry? Stop and ask your body if it has had enough food for now. Constantly stay in touch with your body, especially when you're eating, and listen to what it tells you. When you get to a 5, stop.

When you're in the middle of a meal, it's sometimes hard to tell how close you are to the not hungry level. That's when you can use the rule of three. The rule of three simply means that if you don't know whether you're hungry or not, give yourself permission to have three more bites. Not just any three bites, but the three most delicious bites on the plate. Go for your favorites. Eat the foods that are most appealing and satisfying. Chew every last morsel of flavor out of each of those three bites. Then ask your body again if you have reached not hungry. If you're not getting any signals, the chances are that you're at level 5 and if you continue to eat, you will be feeding your head, not your body.

CONCIOUS EATING

How do most of us eat popcorn at the movies? We really enjoy the first two bites, and then the movie starts. The next thing we know we are at the bottom of the box asking ourselves, "Who ate my popcorn?'' That's unconscious eating—you don't really taste or enjoy the food. Your hand goes from the plate to your mouth and back again of its own accord. You become an automatic eating machine. What if you were very careful about what you ate each day, but every night a little monster slipped into your room after you were asleep and poured food down your throat. You wouldn't think that was very funny, but that has exactly the same effect as unconscious eating. If you're going to eat, savor and appreciate each bite as much as you can.

Greg from Pleasant Hill, California, tells this story about his first conscious meal after the workshop: ''I gathered together all my favorite foods and was planning to sit down to the best meal of my life. I had a nice big New York steak, some green beans with slivered almonds, and a baked potato. I put it all out on the table with nice china and glassware, and I didn't do any of the other things I usually do when I eat. No TV, no magazines. I just ate, cut into the steak, and really savored it. Then I tried a couple of the green beans and they were delicious. Everything was great, but it seemed that it was taking an awfully long time to eat, and I was already starting to get full. About five minutes later my hunger was gone, and I had only eaten half the things on my plate!''

When you're aware of what you're putting into your mouth and enjoying it, you don't need to eat nearly as much. You don't even want to. You're experiencing eating, rather than just shoveling food through a hole in your face. I've found three things that helped me break the transition from unconscious to conscious eating.

*The first is to disconnect the eating machine, which we discussed in "Thin for a Day"—put your fork down BEFORE starting to chew

*The next thing is to stop halfway through the meal, put your fork down, and stop eating completely. Then take a moment to think about what you are going to do after the meal is over and begin to get mentally set to do that.

*Third, estimate how many bites of food it takes you to get to level 5 of not hungry. Sometimes it only takes three to six bites to go from a 4 to a 5. It takes some people only six to nine bites to get from a 3 to a 5 and so on. Don't turn this idea into another diet mentality trick. If you use it, use it only as a way to keep yourself conscious, not to make yourself feel deprived.

*Fourth, write down what and how much you are going to eat BEFORE you eat it. If you find that you cannot finish what you anticipated, go back and reduce the amount you wrote down. If you finish the food on your list and are still hungry, write down how much more you are going to eat, and then begin to eat that.

Writing down what you are going to eat AFTER you eat it is not going to produce the same results. Many times people use writing down what they have eaten as a subtle way to beat themselves up.

When you write down what you are going to eat BEFORE you eat it, you can enjoy the food twice. Once, while looking forward to eating it, and a second time while you are actually eating it.

Look back over the four ideas I just presented and ask yourself these questions. Do naturally thin people do these things? The answer is probably no. Do naturally thin people do some of these things unconsciously? Maybe.

The point is #3 and #4 are definitely crutches. Crutches are fine when your legs are wobbly, but you quickly reach a point where continuing to use them will hold you back more than help you.

STARVING IS OUT

Sometimes when people start to think naturally thin, they overdo it. The feeling of hunger is so new to them, it makes them feel high. They begin to want to feel hungry all the time. Some have gone for days without eating, just trying to see how hungry and high they can get.

The problem with letting yourself get too hungry is that, in the end, you will binge. You're so hungry when you finally do eat, you may never stop. Not only that, but you feel as if you deserve to eat two days' worth of food at one sitting. Again, starving doesn't work because it hooks you back into the Diet Mentality. Food becomes thought of as a reward.

Starving and then going on a binge defeats the purpose of thinking like a naturally thin person. It puts emphasis on food or the lack of it. One way or another it makes food more important than it is. One of the underlying principles of thinking like a naturally thin person is that food isn't all that significant. You eat when you're hungry, enjoy your meals, and stop when the hunger is gone. If you're alternately starving yourself and then going on a binge, your life will still be centered around food.

MASTERING THE CLOCK

You don't have to eat just because it's a certain time of day. Meal times are set up arbitrarily. People in different parts of the world eat at different times of the day. There's nothing sacred or particularly natural about breakfast, lunch, and dinner.

For the next week eat only when you are hungry, as if breakfast, lunch, and dinner didn't exist. When are you hungry? Probably at different times from other people.

Eating by the clock is a good way to fall back into unconscious eating. The clock says noon, so you start putting food into your mouth just because the hands on the clock are pointing up. You don't think about whether you're hungry, or even about what you want to eat. You just move automatically toward food.

Eating because it's time to eat doesn't even have to center around breakfast, lunch, and dinner. You may have a friend with whom you always take your morning coffee break. Each day the two of you go down to the cafeteria or the deli and grab a bite to eat. You do it as a ritual, more out of habit and companionship than out of hunger. Ask yourself whether you want to continue doing that. You can still take breaks with your friend, but you can change the ritual. You might want to take a walk together rather than eat. The important thing is that you don't have to continue doing something just because it is a habit.

Another way you can use time to fool yourself into eating more than you want is by saying, "If I don't eat now, I'll be starving by the time dinner comes." Maybe you will and maybe you won't. Eat what you want now, and let later take care of itself. Your eating habits and patterns will be changing. Let your body develop its own patterns. Avoid preventive eating. Carry an apple or orange around in your pocket if it makes you feel more secure. And who said you had to wait till dinner to eat, anyway? You can eat anytime you are hungry, even in the middle of the afteroon. Don't get caught up in the arbitrary structure of meals. You and your body are in charge, not the clock.

HUNGRY OR THIRSTY?

When I first started eating like a naturally thin person, I discovered something that shocked me. I was in the habit of heading for the kitchen as soon as I sensed messages from my stomach or my mouth that said, "I want something!" Notice that they didn't say, "I'm hungry." They just wanted something.

After I started thinking like a naturally thin person, I'd stop in the middle of the kitchen and ask myself, "At what level of hunger are you now?" Silence. There was no real hunger, just a craving for something.

Then I tried drinking water—a few sips of water—instead of eating food, and about 90% of the time, the craving would go away. As it turned out, I was thirsty, not hungry, but my mind had learned to interpret any kind of craving as a craving for food.

More and more often I found that a drink of water would satisfy my "hunger." If I was still hungry even after drinking the water, I'd have something to eat. But I'd put my hunger to the water test first.

Most of us do not drink enough plain water. Water is one of the most overlooked essential ingredients in our daily food intake. Find water from a source that tastes good to you. Discover which temperature you like it the best and keep a full glass on you desk or near where you spend a lot of time. Get in the habit of drinking water at every chance you get. Make it a part of your naturally thin life.

EXERCISE:

The next time you feel hungry, try drinking water and see if the "hunger" goes away. Were you able to satisfy what you thought was hunger by satisfying your thirst?

Today's date:

TRUST YOUR BODY'S INSTINCTS

Your body knows more than you may think it knows. It's not just some dumb package you wrap yourself in, feed, and drag around from place to place. It's a living entity, with its own way of doing things and its own special kind of knowledge. Think of all the things your body does without your awareness: your heart pumps, your food is digested, air is breathed and assimilated, millions of cells are manufactured and

155

sustained, delicate chemicals are kept in balance, even when you're asleep.

Your body gravitates naturally toward a state of health and comfort and acts without thinking for self–preservation. But you can disrupt the healing of the cut on your finger by picking at it, by interfering with the body's natural processes. In the same way, you can slow down or stop your body's natural progress toward a healthy weight by picking at it mentally. Feeding your head and your emotions rather than your body makes it harder for the body to do its job. Your body may be crying for one thing and being told, "Shut up and eat this." At first you may be a little skeptical or embarrassed. You may go off to a corner and say, "All right, body, what do you want?" You listen and hear nothing.

"See?" you say, "My body doesn't talk to me. It doesn't even have a voice." Listen again. Your body isn't used to your listening to it. Communication may be a bit stilted at first, just as it is with a new friend. But if you listen patiently, you're going to get an answer. In the beginning you might not want to demand a specific food from your body when you ask it what it wants. Instead, you might want to ask it what kind of food would taste good. Go for the substance of the food, the qualities it has.

Give your body a recipe. Does it want something hot or cold? Soft or hard? Salty or sweet? Bland or zippy? Solid or liquid?

156

You might ask your body, "What kind of food would taste really good right now?" And it might answer, "Something crunchy." You can take it from there, asking questions until you get the answer.

"French fries?" you ask.

"No. Too greasy."

"Carrots?"

"No. Too plain. I want something with some zip to it."

"How about an apple fritter?"

"Maybe, but it sounds pretty sweet."

"A plain apple?"

"Yes! That's it."

After a while you don't have to play twenty questions with your body. Just quiet down inside and ask, and it will give you the answer right away. The better listener you become, the more quickly you get your answers.

It's the same with exercise. Sometimes your body will want a lot of it, and sometimes all it will want is a nap. Your body has a life of its own and knows exactly what it needs to sustain that life.

Naturally thin people view their bodies as their friends. They don't have to fight them. They can relax and let their bodies support them.

Are you willing at this moment to let go of your fears and trust your naturally thin body unconditionally?

GET INTO ACTION

"Objects in motion tend to stay in motion. Objects at rest tend to remain at rest."

What if you are stuck? You are not moving forward as a naturally thin person as fast as you would like and you may not even care anymore. What do you do?

Get in motion. Do something and continue doing something until you are moving ahead once more.

Don't stop. Keep doing something. For instance, one lady dropped in on a support meeting at a nationally known weight loss organization. They were moving too slow for her, but at least she was doing something. In this case she was narrowing down the possibilities. She was eliminating options which were not going to work for her.

ABOUT EXERCISE

Kids love to move their bodies. They don't even think of it as work. Exercise is just something that feels good. You were a kid once, remember? Do you recall when you enjoyed that joy in movement?

For most of us, we lost the joy of moving our bodies in school—we were trained to sit still. If we didn't, we risked a poor grade in conduct. After years of such training, we were able to sit for hours and hours without moving. Then came TV—more sitting. And when we gained our weight, we became even more of a spectator and less of a participator. It's time to reverse that downward spiral of inaction. It's predicted that by the year 1997, one-third of the people in this country will be walking, jogging, biking, or roller skating to work. If you live far from work, you'd better start getting in shape now.

Exercise should be a gift you give your body. Listen to your body, and it will tell you when it wants to move around and play. Do exercise that produces the maximum results for you and that you enjoy. Once you get into shape again, exercise will relax you, eliminate stress, and make you look younger and firmer.

Many people exercise as if they're punishing their bodies. When they work out at the health club or gym, they seem to be saying, "Take that! and that!" They look grim and don't seem to be enjoying themselves at all. It doesn't have to be that way.

With exercise, it is usually best to hold yourself back in the beginning. You probably have no idea how out of shape you are. It's better to do too little than too much at first. In fact, even if you cut in half what you think you can do easily, you will probably still be doing too much. Start very slowly. Be lazy. Just do a little today and a little more tomorrow. It takes six weeks to get in shape to start training at full speed. If you start out giving it all you have, you will get sore and tired and want to quit.

Years ago the mother of one of my friends became overweight, then went on a crash diet and lost thirty pounds. The problem was that she didn't look much better than she did before she lost the weight. In those days people assumed that you were either born with a well proportioned body or you weren't. Most people didn't know that they could sculpt their bodies to exactly the shape they wanted.

Behind every curve in your body is a muscle, and how firm and well toned that muscle is determines how nice that curve looks. An attractive, well shaped body is something that most people have to work for, but it shouldn't be painful. Exercising with weights and equipment is by far the fastest and surest way to sculpt your body and get the shape you want.

A few words about jogging: it's great for people who are built for it. The problem is that if you're overweight, your body isn't designed to do this form of exercise very well. Even though your heart and lungs are strengthened, jogging doesn't produce the beautiful, sculptured look that lifting weights does. Most people don't realize that jogging three miles and walking three miles accomplish almost the same benefits. By walking, you burn the same amount of calories, don't have to spend a lot of time warming up, cooling down, and stretching, don't need to buy elaborate jogging shoes, and can fit your exercise more easily into a busy schedule. Instead of having sit-down meetings with my associates, I take them for a walk when we have something to discuss. It adds a relaxed pace to our all-too-hectic lives.

In Europe people walk almost everywhere and often carry canes or walking sticks. When I tried one, I was amazed at how much more enjoyable it made walking. It helps keep your posture straight and tall and isn't a bad crime and dog deterrent either.

"If I chose to exercise, these are the things I will do and when I will start:"

a.

b.

c.

d.

e.

CHEAP EQUIPMENT IS
NOT A BARGAIN

After over thirty years in the health club business, I can share at least one piece of advice with you which could save you ten times the price of this book. Don't buy cheap exercise equipment.

I have talked to thousands of my health club clients who came and joined the club after they had bought some piece of exercise equipment which was used a few times and wound up as a hanging rack gathering dust in some corner. In most cases the piece of equipment was bought "on sale" and was the least expensive model. "Why pay five times as much for what looks like the same thing?" they thought.

The only problem was that when they got the cheap piece of equipment home and began to use it they found that it was not as much fun as they imagined it was going to be and their resolve to "exercise while they watched TV" soon vanished. What happened?

Inexpensive equipment is made cheaply. All the "frills" which give long lasting and smooth performance are eliminated. The problem is that if something is not fun or does not make you feel good when you use it, you will usually not use it for long.

If you are going to buy equipment or join a health club, try it out first. Even though a few of the movements on some of the machines may feel a little awkward at first, make sure that you can learn to enjoy using the machine.

My wife and I have joined two different health clubs. We like both places and exercise more often because we don't get bored going to the same place all of the time.

It is false economy not to get the best quality. In the long run it usually turns out to be the best investment. The best piece of equipment will be the one that you use often.

The worst thing about buying cheap equipment is that it delays you in doing something that you were fired up to do. Instead of moving you forward, you wind up wasting your money and failing once again to do something that you promised yourself that you would do.

CHAPTER 11

MAKING THE ATTITUDE TRANSITION

It is primitive thinking to believe that if you deprive yourself from eating exactly what you want for long enough, that you will lose your weight and keep it off. It is out–of–date thinking.

If you are going to see a permanent shift in your weight or your eating, the shift is going to come from the questions that you begin to ask yourself.

If you get stuck, you are asking the wrong questions. The answers don't matter very much if the wrong questions are asked. The power comes from the questions.

What are some powerful questions that you could be asking? What diet should I go on? What shouldn't I eat? What should I eat to lose weight? All of these are diet mentality questions and these questions will keep giving you the same results you have achieved in the past. Losing and gaining. Losing and gaining.

In order to have a breakthrough with your weight and eating, you are going to have to begin a new way of thinking. A new way of looking at old problems.

The main thing is to be patient with yourself, give yourself plenty of time, and leave room for error. Expect your life to be different and don't be surprised when people treat you differently. Keep your sense of humor. I've never met anyone who became naturally thin by being grim and serious.

IT'S OK TO HAVE FEELINGS

Most of the eating habits we've talked about have an emotional dimension. In some cases the specific purpose of overeating is trying to get rid of feelings, to make them go away by literally stuffing them down with food.

Stuffing feelings down with food is a bad game to play, a game that's difficult to win. You're always going to have feelings, both positive and negative, and if you head for the refrigerator every time you start to have what you consider to be an uncomfortable emotion, you're going to get very heavy in a hurry. If, on the other hand, you can unhook food from your emotions, you accomplish two important things:

* Your weight is no longer dependent on how you feel;

* You can bring your emotions to the surface, experience them, and do something about them.

You can't deal with something you won't let yourself see or experience. It's like playing Blind Man's Bluff. When you let emotions like sadness, loneliness, anger, fear, or grief come to the surface and allow yourself to experience them fully, you'll find that most of the time they dissipate of their own accord. Some people are afraid that if they let their feelings surface, those feelings will stay around forever. Just the opposite is true.

Gail, of Aspen, said, "The first week I couldn't believe it. I was crying all the time. One afternoon I realized that I was crying about my mother, who'd died the year before. I'd never let myself feel the grief then and had started stuffing it down with food. After a week the tears just stopped, and I feel better now than I have in the entire year since my mother passed away."

Some people find it useful to set aside five minutes each day when they can really get into some particular feeling—sadness, fear, or pity, for example. They sit down and allow themselves to feel as sad, afraid, or sorry for themselves as possible for the full five minutes. When they are finished, the sadness, fear, or pity is usually gone.

Keeping your emotions down is like trying to hold back a dam. Sooner or later, if the pressure isn't released, the dam is going break, overflow, or come out at a place where it can't be controlled. And when it does, the problems your feelings cause will be far worse than the five minutes you spent letting yourself feel those emotions.

We have emotional appetites as well as physical appetites, and those emotional appetites can't be satisfied with food. Emotions, both positive and negative, are a healthy part of life. Grief and joy come up the same tunnel in us. To the degree we suppress either one, we automatically suppress the other. Your feelings are a part of you. Trying to make them go away only causes them to torment you.

Ellen shared at a Diets Don't Work Weekend Workshop in San Francisco, "Being assertive is hard for me. Rather than making a direct request of someone to give me exactly what I want, I swallow the request...Literally." Ellen's problem didn't get resolved until she stopped putting food in her mouth to deal with her discomfort.

The side benefit, of course, is that you begin to learn to handle your feelings quickly and easily. You actually may start to enjoy and encourage your feelings to come to the surface.

EXERCISES (7 minutes)

1. "These are the worst things that could happen if I let my emotions come to the surface":

a.

b.

c.

d.

e.

RELATING TO OTHERS
AS A THIN PERSON

When you first start living like a thin person, people are going to be surprised. They may also be upset. They may think you've gone completely crazy. When you order a pizza, they may look at you suspiciously and say, "I thought you were on a diet?" You can just turn to them and smile. "Yes. A Pizza diet." You can have a lot of fun if you tell them how much weight you've already lost and that you found this great diet in the book called *DIETS STILL DON'T WORK.*

Many of them won't have read this book, so they won't know what you're up to. Even when you explain, they may have some of the same doubts and concerns you did when you first considered living like a naturally thin person. They may think it won't work.

Some people think that anything worthwhile can be gained only through deprivation, suffering, and agony. They may find it hard to believe that your way can be so simple and easy and still produce results. Give it time. When they start to see the pounds and inches disappear, they'll believe. Till then you just have to recognize that your disbelieving friends and relatives are relating to you as the fat person they knew in the past, not the naturally thin person you are now becoming. You may have to establish a whole new relationship with them.

Whenever you begin a new relationship with yourself, you have to start a new relationship with others, too.

Carol, who lives in southern California, told me that she used to go out with her eating buddies at least once a week. They went to restaurants or buffets and overate. After the weekend workshop, she realized that she did not enjoy overeating. Spending time with her friends, even if she didn't join the overeating, was not fun for her any longer. She was afraid that if she continued to hang around an environment of unconscious eating, she would soon be sucked into overeating once again. She sat her friends down and used the withhold technique from Chapter 9. It worked beyond her wildest dreams. They asked if they could join and support her effort to become naturally thin. They all bought copies of *DIETS DON'T WORK* and used their once a week get–together to work through the book chapter by chapter. Their overeating group has now turned into a *DIETS DON'T WORK* support group and they are all losing weight and supporting each other in being naturally thin.

Maybe you want to surround yourself with as many people as you can to support you in being a naturally thin person. Maybe you want to do it alone. You may want a lot of verbal encouragement or maybe you want the people around you to just shut up and leave you alone. Maybe you want to eat out all the time or you may want to eat at home. Maybe you want all of your friends and family to read this book. Maybe you just don't want to discuss anything to do with weight for two months. It's up to you. There's no right way to become naturally thin. You have to see what will work for you and what ways of relating to others will support you best. You are the only one with the answers.

You may run into some resistance. Have you ever run across a person who seems to think they know better than you do about what's best for you? Do you need to tell them what you want and don't want from them? If they really are committed to helping you, have them read *DIETS STILL DON'T WORK* and be your partner in losing weight. Each time they see you, before they can ask you about your weight, ask them if they have read the book yet? Sometimes it will be uncomfortable, but one thing is for sure— you'll find out who really supports you.

Enthusiastically concentrate on living and eating like a naturally thin person. Soon you'll have a lot of people wanting to join you and have the results you are producing.

EXERCISE (5 minutes)

"These are the specific requests I will make of people to support me when I start living like a naturally thin person:" (Ask for a specific promise. Make sure the promise is for a specific period of time or by a certain time. "Will you promise to...?")

a.

b.

c.

d.

e.

Go back over the above requests and include how long you want the promise to be for ("for the rest of today?") or by when you want the promise completed ("by this Friday at 6 P.M.?").

Make sure when you get promises that you hold the persons accountable. Follow up with them. Graciously thank and acknowledge these persons when they do what they said they would do. If they break their promises, ask them if you understood their promises correctly. If they broke their word to you, gently acknowledge that. Give them your permission to revoke their promises if they do not want to keep them. They may want to remake the promises or renegotiate a promise that they can be counted on to keep.

GOOD-BYE DEPRIVATION

Most people automatically want to eat more of anything they don't think they can have. If certain foods are off limits to you, they become more tantalizing. If you say to yourself, "No more candy. No more Oreos," your mind will become preoccupied with just those things.

You'll be playing right back into the Diet Mentality, setting up rules for yourself that can only have one of two results:

* You eat them anyway and feel guilty;

* You don't eat them, but you feel deprived. You're a martyr, nailed to the cross. You go around with a huge burden on your shoulders, heaving enormous sighs.

That isn't what being a naturally thin person is about. Being naturally thin is about enjoying life more and ending your preoccupation with food. Part of the joy of living like a naturally thin person is that you can eat exactly what you want to. It's also one of the guidelines. If you're depriving yourself, you're thinking like a fat person, not like a naturally thin person.

Your body is going to want certain foods, and it's going to go after them with a vengeance. Assume your body tells you it wants asparagus with hollandaise sauce. "Hollandaise sauce!" you say. "You must be crazy. Do you know how many calories and fat are in hollandaise? Why don't you have this nice lettuce leaf instead." But if you eat the lettuce leaf, the little voice inside you will still be whispering, "Asparagus with hollandaise. Asparagus with hollandaise." So you say, "Here. If you have to be bad, eat these oatmeal cookies." You eat the oatmeal cookies, thinking surely that will shut up the voice. If you stuff him/her full of food, he/she won't want anything, much less asparagus with hollandaise.

But you still hear the whisper. Finally, you get to the point where you just can't do without asparagus with hollandaise. You go to the kitchen and fix it, and finally your body smiles and relaxes. Now you have all the calories in the asparagus and hollandaise, plus the calories in the oatmeal cookies. You would have been better off just eating the asparagus in the first place.

There may come a time when you want to make certain foods off limits. For instance, some people say that every time they drink coffee, they feel terrible. If that happens, you don't want to moan, "Oh, no. I can never drink coffee again!" Give yourself permission to drink it and allow yourself to feel exactly what happens. You will probably reach a point where you don't want it. The pain you go through when you drink coffee, or whatever it is for you, will be worse than the pain of not having it. Your body will rebel against that food, not because it shouldn't have it, but because it doesn't want it.

Your body's wants and needs may change, especially as the pounds start to go away. Next week it may be fine for you to eat the food your body didn't want last week. Stay attuned to your body, listening for the changes that are taking place.

And don't deprive yourself. Give your body what it wants. That's one of the hallmarks of eating like a naturally thin person.

THE SCALE CAN BE YOUR ENEMY

You get up in the morning and step onto the scale. (You always weigh yourself in the morning because that way you haven't had a chance to eat in seven or eight hours.) One of three things has happened: you've gained weight, you've lost weight, or you've stayed the same.

If you've lost weight, you're ahead of the game and can afford to cheat a little. If you've gained weight, you may feel angry or depressed. If you've stayed the same, it looks as if what you're doing is for nothing. What's the likely response to any of those three responses? To eat, of course. The scale can actually be a trigger to overeat.

The scale can work against you in other ways, too. Aside from the fact that it's very difficult to find a scale that's accurate all the time, using a scale can lead you to the misconception that how you look is determined by what you weigh. That's not always true.

The scale is one of the most inaccurate ways to measure fat loss that I know of. Your goal is to have your body look exactly the way you want it to, and the scale doesn't reflect that. If you want to use something to measure your progress, a tape measure is better than a scale. Or use your clothes. Pounds and inches are not the same. The scale may not say that you're losing weight, but if your clothes are getting looser, you know you're making progress.

A pound of fat is about twice as large as a pound of muscle, yet it takes fewer calories to sustain. In other words, the more fat you have in proportion to muscle, the less food your body will need. The more muscular you are, the more food your body will need. That's one reason you can watch someone who is thin and beautifully toned sit down and eat a huge meal without gaining weight. You can't figure out where they're putting it, but it's all going to feed their muscles.

Furthermore, after you get to be twenty–six years old, your body starts playing a trick on you. It takes half a pound of muscle each year and turns it into fat. It's called aging. With each year that goes by, another half a pound of what used to be muscle is now fat.

That's not so bad, you say, half a pound a year. But they add up. By the time you're thirty–six years old, you have five more pounds of fat on your body than you did when you were twenty-six, even if you weigh the same. The clothes that fit you then won't fit you now.

Have you ever had an old pair of slacks that are finally back in style and sent them to the cleaners expecting to be able to wear them again? But even though you still weigh the same, they no longer fit you. The cleaners seem to have shrunk them. But that's not what's happened. You just have five more pounds of fat than you did before, and it's bigger than the muscle it has replaced.

It's a cruel trick, but our bodies do that to us. It's one of the many reasons scales aren't really the best way to measure your progress.

If you have to get on the scale, treat it like a horoscope. Only believe it if it gives you good news.

EXERCISE   (3 minutes)

"This is what would happen if I didn't get on a scale for:"

a. A week:

b. Two weeks:

c. A month:

If you weighed yourself less often, a scale might even become your friend. Look at two pounds of hamburger meat or two pounds of butter the next time you go to the store. Could you acknowledge how much two pounds is when it is concentrated in one lump?

What if someone told you that you could reduce the overall size of your body by the amount of space that two pounds of hamburger takes up by eating like a naturally thin person for one month? Would you get excited? What if you could lose that much mass in two weeks? How about if you lost that much in just one week, would you begin to worry that you were losing weight too fast?

The scale can motivate you and validate that you are living your life like a naturally thin person. Just don't give it any more power over your life than you give your toaster. If you can't do that, make your bathroom seem larger. Throw your scale away.

KEEPING A JOURNAL OR DIARY

Many people who read *DIETS DON'T WORK* told me that they found a lot of value from keeping a daily record of their thoughts. Writing out the conversations they were having in their heads made it clear that the naturally thin part of themselves was alive and kicking. The thin part didn't win all of the battles, but they could tell from reading back over their journals that the naturally thin part was getting stronger every day.

There are some very good books about journal writing at your local book store. If you need help in finding one, send me a self-addressed, stamped envelope. Let me know what you are looking to accomplish and I will send you a list of appropriate books.

A journal or a diary keeps the naturally thin voice inside of you strong and clear. Don't let it fade. The Diet Mentality voice is just waiting for you to back slide.

IMAGING

All the books on success tell us that people who have clear goals and think of them all of the time almost always wind up attaining their goals. People who have vague goals and don't think of them very often seldom attain their goals. How do you make sure you are going to reach your goal of being naturally thin?

To make sure you wind up naturally thin, create a clear mental image of exactly the way you want to look and hold that image in your mind as often as possible. Begin to think of yourself as already naturally thin from the moment you open your eyes in the morning until you are falling asleep at night. Walk, talk, shower, work, exercise, write in your daily journal, and eat as if you were already naturally thin. As you go through the day, think the same thoughts and feel the same feelings you would have if you had already reached your goal.

Practicing being naturally thin is a good strategy for several reasons. First, creating a mental image of what you want to look like and beginning to feel those feelings and think naturally thin thoughts will tell your mind exactly where to take you.

Second, you don't know exactly what you're going to find at the end of the rainbow. If you've been overweight for some time, you may not have any idea of what you're going to look like if you lose your weight. You aren't even ready for the way other people will relate to you as you begin to act like a naturally thin person.

If you were exactly where you wanted to be right now, and you took off all your clothes and stood in front of a mirror and saw your perfect body, would you recognize it? If you don't have a clear, vivid picture of what it would look like, take some time to create one.

Look in magazines and find arms, thighs, calves, stomachs, hips, feet, and hands that look like parts of your naturally thin body. These parts can have clothes on or not. Paste them up on one of the pages of your daily journal and look at your naturally thin body everyday. The best times to plant this picture in your mind are the first thing in the morning, before you exercise, and just before you turn out the lights at night. If you loved someone, looking at an attractive picture of them a couple of times a day wouldn't seem strange, would it? Maybe all that you need to do to become naturally thin is to fall in love with the most important person in the world and love their rear end off. . . literally.

EXERCISES

1. Find or go buy some magazines. Go through them and begin to cut out parts which resemble parts of your naturally thin body. Put these pieces in an envelope.

2. Take the pieces of your naturally thin body out and spread them on a page in your daily journal. Once you get enough of the perfect pieces to create the image and feeling of your naturally thin body, paste them permanently on the page.

3. For at least the next six weeks, look at the picture of your naturally thin body at least twice a day.

WHO'S CRAZY?

One of the greatest definitions of insanity I ever heard was quoted by Werner Erhard, creator of THE FORUM, a two weekend course about the creation of possibility where little or none presently exists in every area of a person's life. Werner said, "Insanity is doing the SAME thing over and over and over and over, hoping for a DIFFERENT result."

The world is full of insane fat people. They continue to do the same thing over and over and over and over, hoping for a different result.

I invite you to take on the vision of ending weight and overeating as a problem for everyone by the year 2000 A.D.. The biggest step you could take is to start with yourself. If you wish to do more, I will be forever grateful. Please write and share your promises, visions, and accomplishments with me.

BOB SCHWARTZ
P.O. BOX 2866
HOUSTON, TEXAS 77252-2866

Chapter 12

WHAT NOW? QUESTIONS AND ANSWERS

Q. I am so hard on myself. I seem to be constantly beating myself up. I keep expecting myself to be perfect and to be a lot further along than I am.

A. THE CURE TO BEATING YOURSELF UP. Ask yourself if you can love yourself for what you just did, thought, or felt. Let's say that you get in a hurry and start getting impatient and you realize what you are doing. Ask yourself, can you (the naturally thin you) love yourself for doing that and let it go?

Whatever you did or did not do is not the end of the world. What do you want to do now? What result do you want now?

Give yourself permission to be human. You are not a machine. You are not perfect all of the time. You never will be and to expect perfection at all times from yourself is just setting yourself up to lose.

You are doing the best that you can for now. Next time will be different and you will be able to do better next time. Enjoy the journey. Having as much pleasure as possible is your new job. Lighten up. You are becoming naturally thin. It's working! Once you reach your goal, this is what the journey you took will have looked like.

Look to see where you are now and recall all the effort you had to go through to get here. At times did it ever look like you were on the wrong path? Well? Here you are, aren't you? You made it this far or you wouldn't be reading this book, would you?

Q. I have been making baby promises and keeping them, but I am, as you predicted, starting to get bored. My baby promises are fine, but they produce baby results. Can I begin to swing out now and make larger promises? What do I do if I miss?

A. If keeping your word, no matter what, has become important to you, you can begin to make bigger promises. Do everything in your power to accomplish your promise. If for any reason you fail, here is what to do.

1. Acknowledge that you broke your promise. Repeat your promise exactly the way you made it and say exactly how you broke it. "I said that I would follow the four rules for eating like a naturally thin person all day today. I followed them exactly at breakfast and lunch, but at dinner I ate until I was a 7."

2. Repair any damage that you have caused by breaking your promise. Ask yourself, what can you do to make up for breaking your promise? If you shared your promise with **anyone** else, admit to that person right away that you broke your promise and ask what you should do to make it up.

3. Make a new promise that you will keep. You need to be a little cautious now. Make sure that you are committed to keeping this new promise and that you will not miss.

4. Forgive yourself for breaking your word and get busy on your new promise.

Q. Are there any *DIETS STILL DON'T WORK* support groups around the country and how can I get into one?

A. Yes, there are support groups. Send me your name, address, and phone number plus a self-addressed stamped envelope and I will let you know of groups in your area.

The easiest way to be in a *DIETS STILL DON'T WORK* support group is to form one yourself. If you want details on how to go about setting one up, let me know.

Support groups have been found to be very valuable in every stage of the naturally thin life. Surround yourself with support so thick you cannot help but reach your weight loss and eating goals.

DEVELOPING
INNER-CENTERED REALITY

What happens now? Let's say you've already worked through all the obstacles that were standing in your way, and you've firmly resolved to go out into the world and think like a naturally thin person for the rest of you life. You accept and love yourself and know that it's only a matter of time before you get a naturally thin body to match your naturally thin thinking.

Then tomorrow you get up and the first person you see looks you up and down and she says, "You know, my aunt was just as fat as you are, and she found this great diet..." What do you do? Punch her out and head for the deli?

There's a whole world out there that hasn't yet given up on diets. Deep down everyone knows that diets aren't the answer, but they're still hanging on, digging those fingernails into dieting even though they're slipping. They don't want to admit they are wrong.

A lot of people think you can't eat exactly what you want and still lose weight. What they don't consider is that you're eating only when you're hungry and stopping when your hunger is gone. Those people won't understand that you're eating to feed your hunger and not your feelings. They're probably used to relating to you the way you were before.

You just have to know that you're doing what works for you. Keep focused on what you're doing and keep putting one foot in front of the other.

Can you honestly say at this moment that you have chosen and are committed to live the rest of your life as a naturally thin person?

Yes:

No:

Not yet:

Today's Date:

Time:

BREATHING SPACE

You may want to give yourself a little breathing space. I've found that it takes about four weeks to break the old habits, another four weeks to get established in the new ones, and at least another four before they start to become automatic.

At some point during that first week, you may find yourself eating for your old reasons. This moment is important. The key to moving through it successfully is not to beat yourself up. Just tell the truth about what you did, recognize that you forgot about being a naturally thin person, and be more aware of the potential danger the next time. You'll slip again. That's normal. The important thing is to pick yourself up, gently dust yourself off, and re-establish your sense of being a naturally thin person.

The pattern of three four–week cycles is just a guideline. It may take you one week or one day or nine months. Just remember not to be too hard on yourself—it may take longer than you think.

EXERCISES (6 minutes)

1. "These are the ways I might be inclined to beat myself up if I stop thinking like a naturally thin person:"

a.

b.

c.

d.

e.

f.

g.

h.

2. "These are the antidotes, the things I will do to stop if I start to beat myself up:"

a.

b.

c.

d.

e.

f.

g.

h.

START ON YOUR GOALS

Make a list of everything you can imagine that you might want. A wish list. Don't worry about how you are going to get or achieve your wishes. Just look in a mirror and keep asking yourself over and over, "If you could have anything that you wanted, what would it be?"

Make sure that you are willing to do what it takes to have those things, but don't edit what thoughts come to you. Just write them down and ask yourself that question over and over again until the next thought comes to you or until you run dry. After each wish is written down, ask yourself what date would be the right date for you to have that wish become a reality. (Use more paper if necessary.)

Some people may keep weight around as a problem because a part of them is afraid that if that problem went away, they would have nothing to do. Their lives would become boring. To avoid that trap, begin to work on your goals. There will be plenty to do, as you'll see when you start working on your list.

You may not think you can possibly accomplish some of the goals on your list until you're actually naturally thin. Those are the best ones to start on now. Doing them will force you to think of yourself as a naturally thin person and reinforce your new points of view.

You will see again that becoming a naturally thin person isn't just about losing weight. It's a way to live your life. When those goals start to happen and your life starts to be the way you want it to be, you'll be amazed how quickly you'll lose interest in food.

EXERCISES (10 minutes)

1. What is the first goal you're going to work on?

2. What is the first step you need to take to accomplish that goal?

3. When are you going to take that first step?

4. Make a game plan for thinking like a naturally thin person. "When I wake up in the morning, I will . . ."

"At 9:00 A.M., I will. . ."

"At noon, I will. . ."

"At 6:00 P.M., I will. . ."

"At 9:00 P.M., I will. . ."

"Before I go to bed, I will..."

"I FEEL FAT...SO I EAT!"

In almost every conversation that I have with people I work with, they all say that one of their problems is that when they feel fat...they eat. This is the most common form of what I call "beating yourself up."

This compulsion to beat yourself up by eating probably comes over you at two main times.

1. WHEN YOU HAVE OVEREATEN: You feel bloated, swollen, ashamed, angry, disappointed, and hopeless. You want to strike out at someone and the person easiest to hit is you. You pick up the nearest food and say "Take that and that and that!"

The cure for this one is to take some kind of positive action. Go do something that moves you forward as a naturally thin person. Sometimes all you have to do is to forgive yourself and promise to begin to act naturally thin from that moment on. Another thing you can do is to whip out your diary and write about what just happened to you and what you are going to do about it.

2. YOU ARE LOOKING INTO THE MIRROR:

Are you looking for things to like about your body? No! You look for what is wrong with you. Your attention is focused only on the bad parts You keep reminding yourself that you are

194

disappointed with your body. What you are doing is like going out into your garden and only looking at the weeds.

From now on, everytime you look in the mirror, I want you to practice looking only and specifically for parts you like.

If there is an area on your body that you can find absolutely nothing good about, even if you bend over backwards, pass by it quickly and go on to the next area. Keep reminding yourself that you are looking for parts to like.

I know this will probably be hard for you, especially if you have spent years looking and complaining about those parts that you don't like.

The reason I am asking you to focus only on what you like is because: WHATEVER YOU PUT YOUR ATTENTION ON WILL EXPAND. If you put your attention on what you don't like or don't want, you will get more of that. If you focus on what is good about you, you will create more good things. Besides, why should you do something nice, like losing weight, for someone that you don't like?

Begin to concentrate on what you are doing that is working. Acknowledge yourself every chance you get. If you don't like something...fix it. If you can't fix it, learn to love it. Get into action and make it happen.

FALLING IN LOVE

There is only one person in the world you can be absolutely, positively sure you'll be living with for the rest of your life...yourself. Your relationship with everyone else on earth comes out of your relationship with yourself. To the extent that you love yourself and recognize the good qualities about you, you'll love others and recognize the best parts of them.

Up to this point there has been a big obstacle in the way of your falling in love with yourself. You saw it every time you looked in the mirror. You may have judged and criticized yourself and found it hard to love any part of the person you saw. Now you have the means to replace that negative attention with positive attention. You have the tools to begin a new life and a new relationship with that person in the mirror whenever you choose. It may take some discipline, but it's a positive discipline rather than a negative one because you're facing rather than avoiding the real issue.

The discipline you'll need is nothing more than remembering to think of yourself as the person you want to be, the naturally thin person. That person already exists. He or she will be your lifelong companion just for the asking. It can be a life and a relationship filled with support, love, and happiness.

You can have more joy, peace, and accomplishment in your life than you ever dreamed possible. You can end weight as a problem in your life forever—today.

It's a simple choice. . . to think like a naturally thin person or to think like a fat person. All it takes is commitment and permission from yourself to let yourself be whichever you choose. You can get on with the rest of your life. You can start to let the joy, peace, and sense of accomplishment you feel spread out into the rest of the world.

"This is how I would describe my commitment to live as a naturally thin person for the rest of my life:"

"My vision is the end of weight as a problem for everyone by the year 2000 A.D.."

Today's date:

Signed:

I recommend that you go back and read this book over and if your answers to the questions change, write down what the changes are. Do this five more times or until the idea of being naturally thin is like second nature to you.

If you have not also read my first book, *DIETS DON'T WORK*, I recommend that you read it now. It contains some of the same basic information found in this book, but it has other information and questions that you will find supportive and useful. It will not hurt you to hear some of this information more than once. Your life is going to change for the better. Many people assisted in putting on the Diets Don't Work Weekend Workshops and asked to be taught how to lead Diets Don't Work support groups in order to stay in a naturally thin environment. *DIETS DON'T WORK* and *DIETS*

STILL DON'T WORK are easy ways to keep the naturally thin conversations alive in your thinking until they take root.

DIETS DON'T WORK and *DIETS STILL DON'T WORK* are available at your local bookstore. Call ahead to check their availability. If the book store has sold out, call the publisher at 1-800-227-1152 and order the book for $9.95 plus $2 shipping with your credit card or send a check for $11.95 to: Breakthru Publishing, P.O. Box 2866, Houston, Texas 77252-2866.

If you are an adult, I also recommend that you read my other book, *THE ONE HOUR ORGASM*, which is based on the research of Dr. W. Victor Baranco of More University. The information in *THE ONE HOUR ORGASM* has proven to be very useful for anyone who is losing weight and becoming more attractive.

THE ONE HOUR ORGASM contains adult sex information which will improve your present relationship and sex life or prepare you for a committed relationship in the future.

You may order *THE ONE HOUR ORGASM* through your local bookstore or by calling 1-800-227-1152.

"IT AIN'T OVER UNTIL THE NATURALLY THIN LADY SINGS!"

Bob Schwartz

CHECK WHICH INFORMATION YOU WOULD
LIKE TO RECEIVE:

___Having a Diets Don't Work Weekend
Workshop in your area or traveling to one.

___Ordering Diets Don't Work Audio tapes
featuring Bob Schwartz.

___Renting or purchasing a Diets Don't Work
Video (VHS) featuring Bob Schwartz.

___Having Bob Schwartz, Lecturer & Humorist
speak at your convention or meeting.

___Ordering 12 or more books for a quantity
discount price.

___Information about making an appointment
for private or family consulting by phone or in
person with Bob Schwartz or his staff.

___Setting up Diets Don't Work weekly support
group meetings in your area.

___Being trained to lead Diets Don't Work
workshops in your area.

___Setting up television or radio interviews
with Bob Schwartz on your local or national
talk show programs.

___ Ordering the Diets Don't Work "Breakthru"
Game.

___Information about ordering *THE ONE HOUR
ORGASM*

Call (713) 522-7660 or send a self-addressed and stamped envelope* to:

DIETS DON'T WORK INFORMATION P.O. Box 2866, HOUSTON, TEXAS (77252–2866)

*PLEASE include a separate sheet with your name, address, and phone number.

Other books by Breakthru Publishing:

*DIETS DON'T WORK!...

The Secrets of Losing Weight Without Dieting.

*THE ONE HOUR ORGASM...

What Your Parents Never Knew or Taught You About Sex And Relationships. Based on the work of Dr. Victor Baranco of More University.

*OFF THE PEDESTAL...

Transforming the Business of Medicine.

Order through your local bookstore or call 1-713-522-7660 and order direct with your credit card.